Surgical Challenges in the Management of Liver Disease

Edited by Georgios Tsoulfas

Published in London, United Kingdom

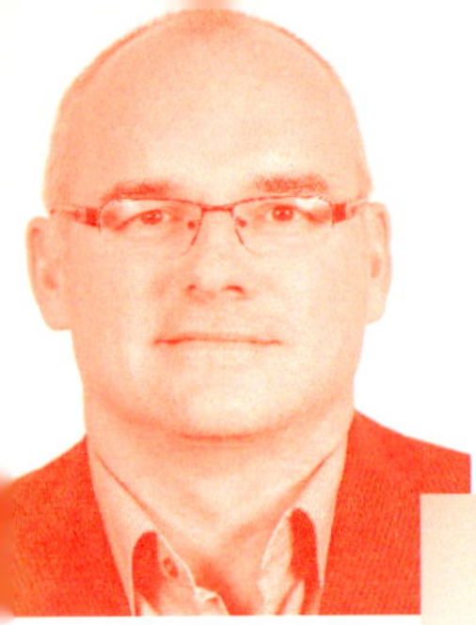
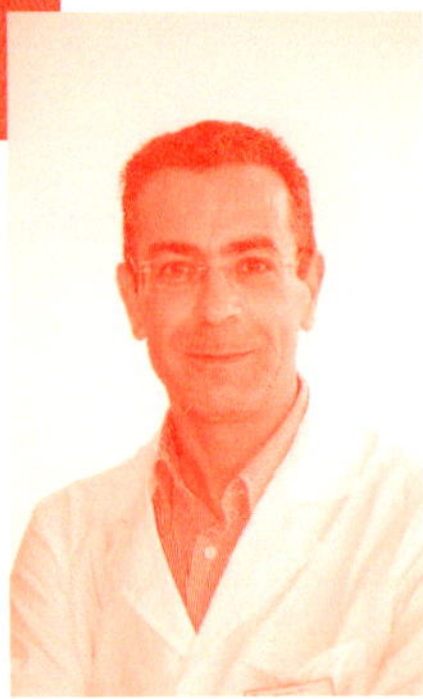
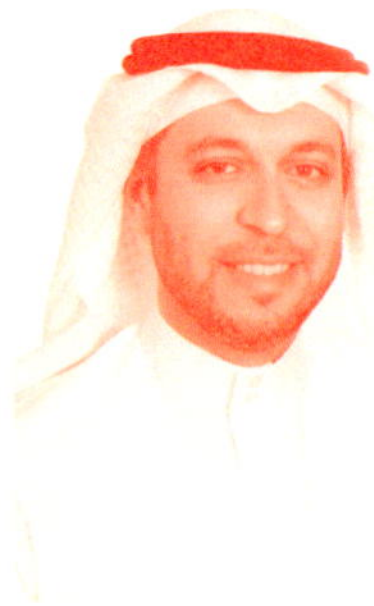
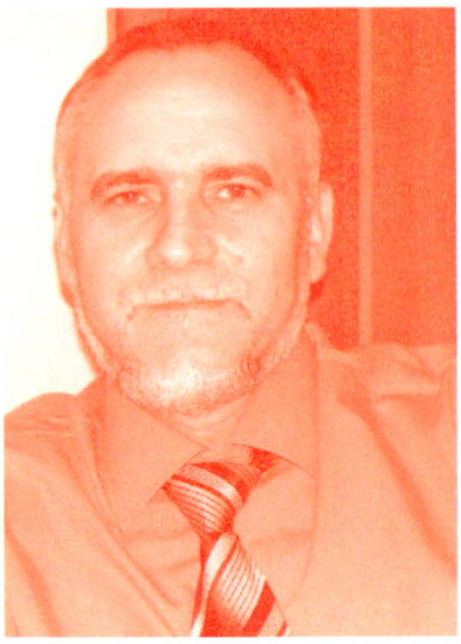
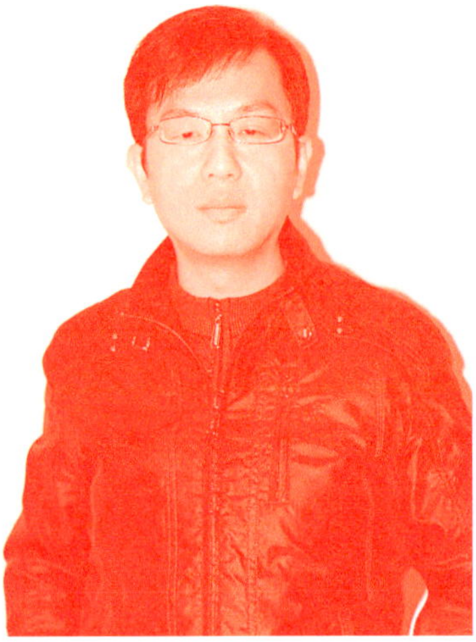
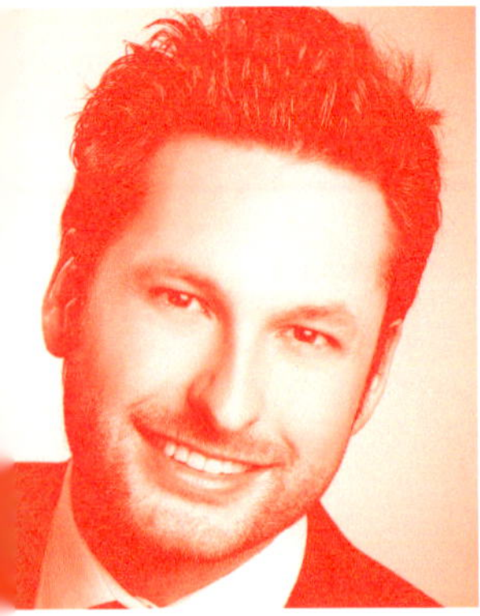
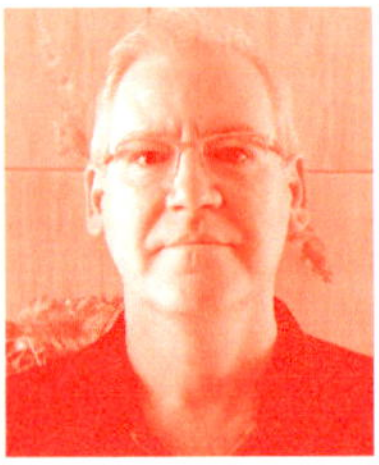

IntechOpen

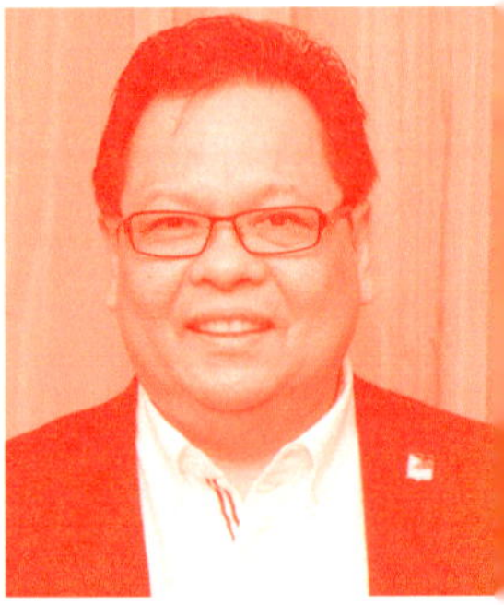
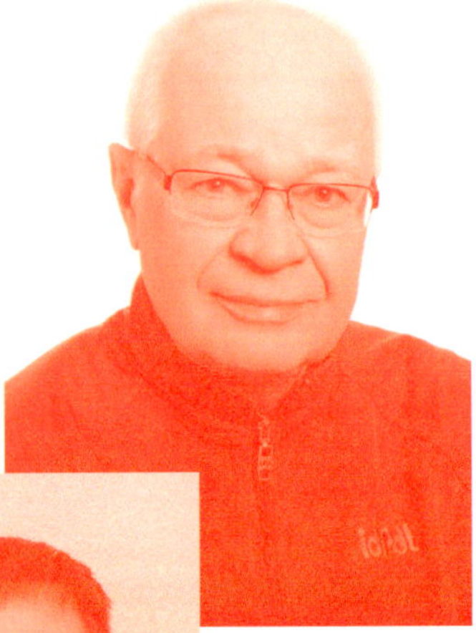
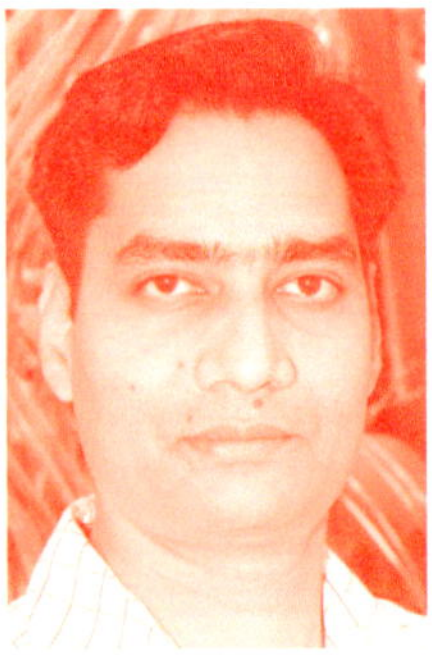
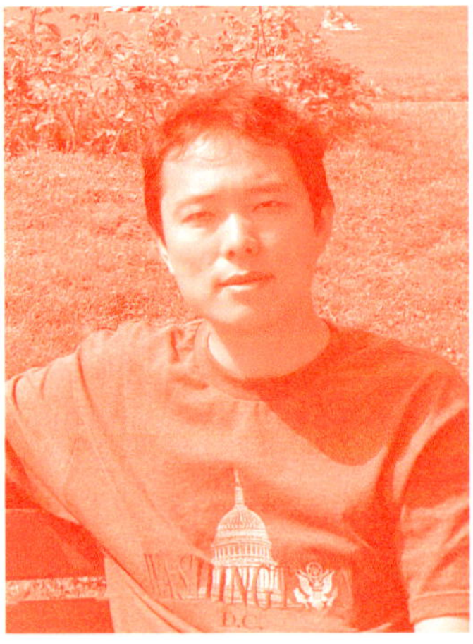
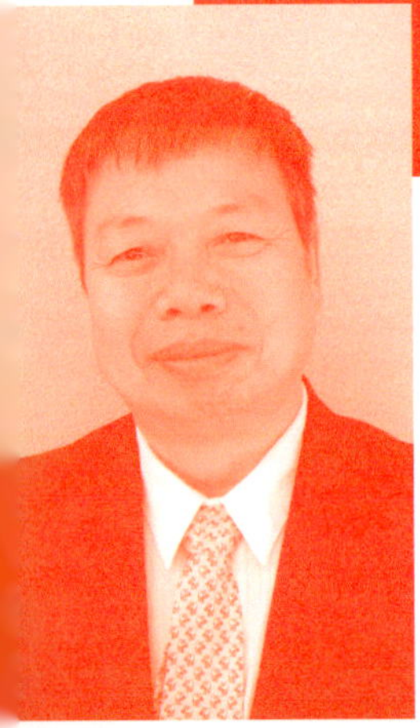
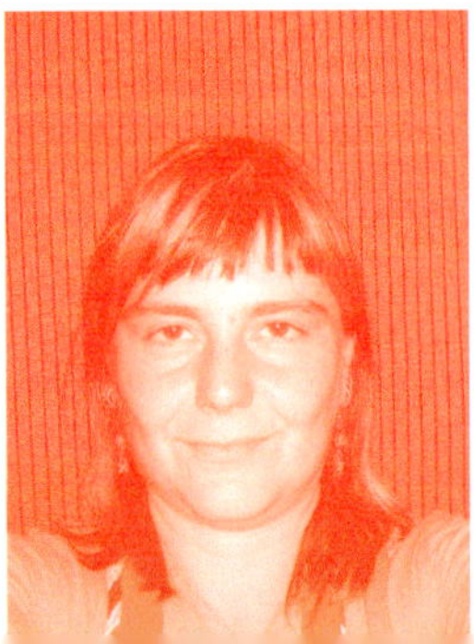

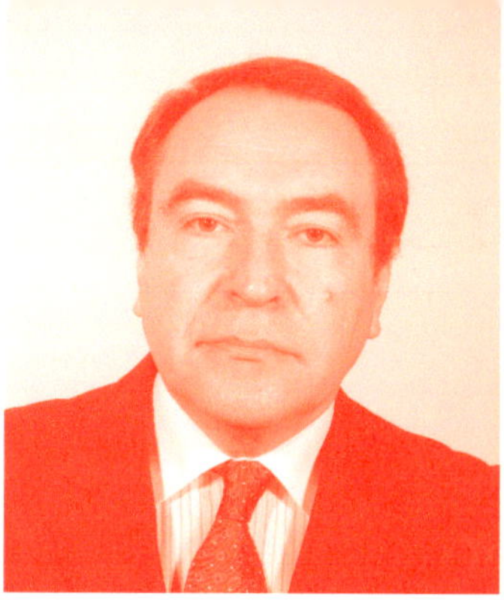
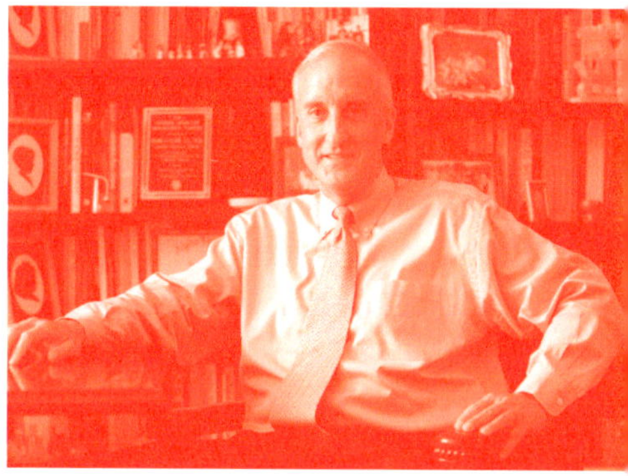
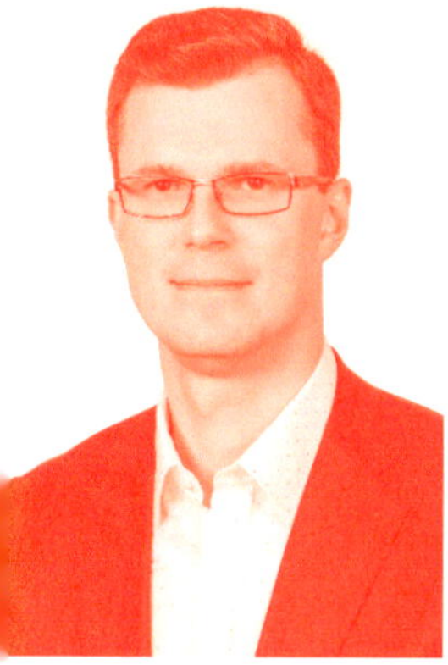
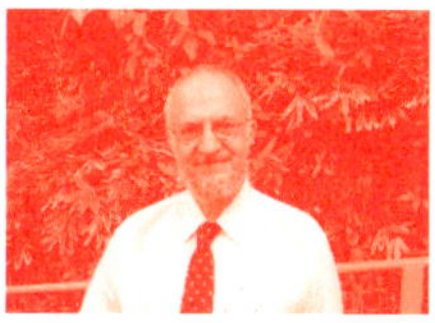
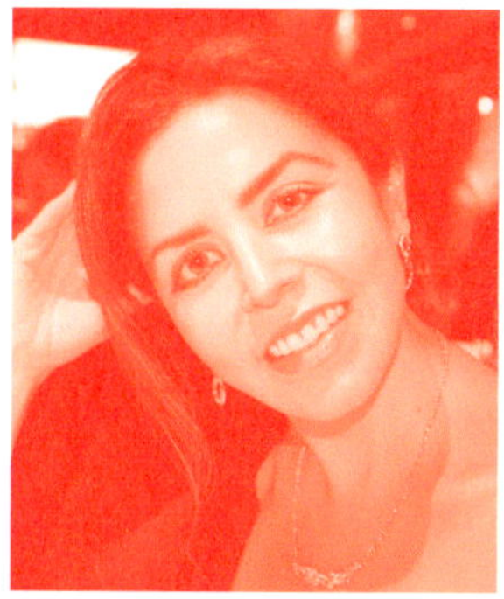

Supporting open minds since 2005

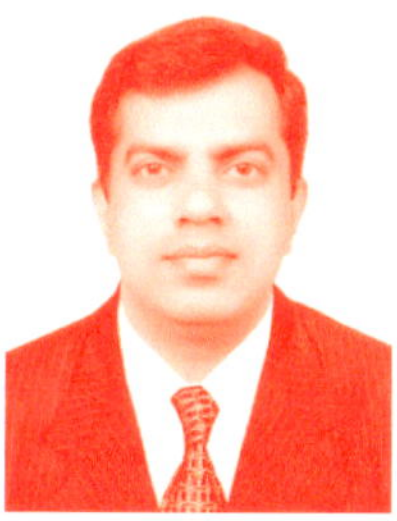
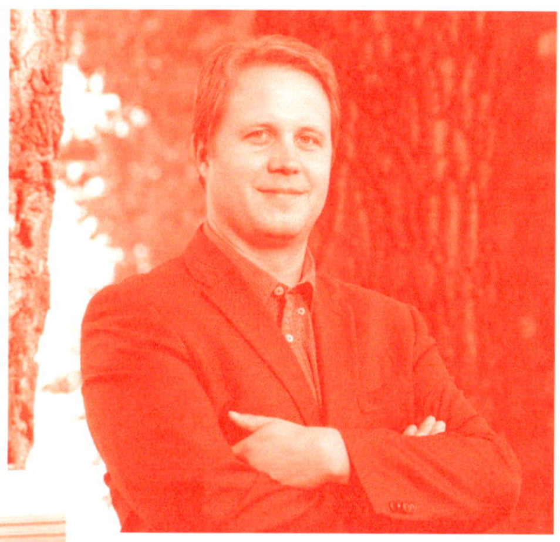
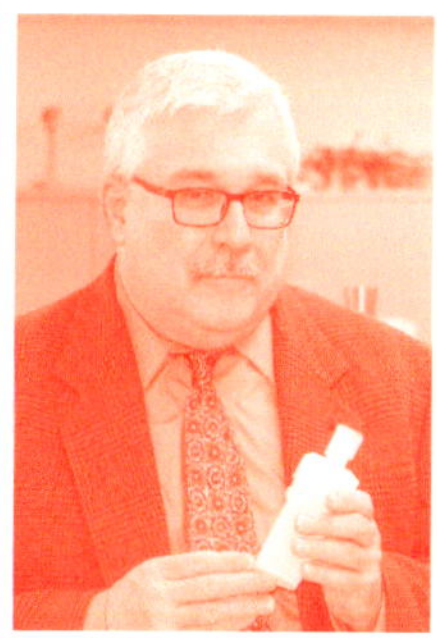
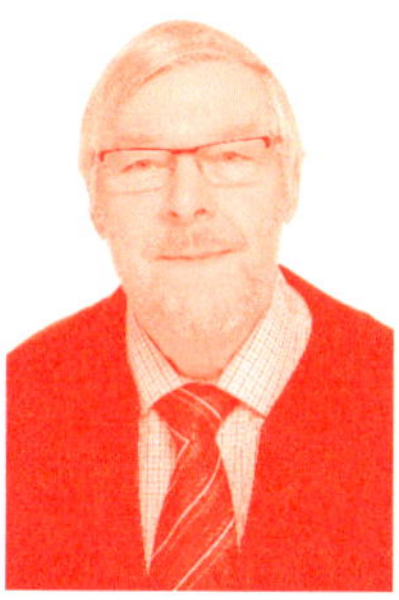
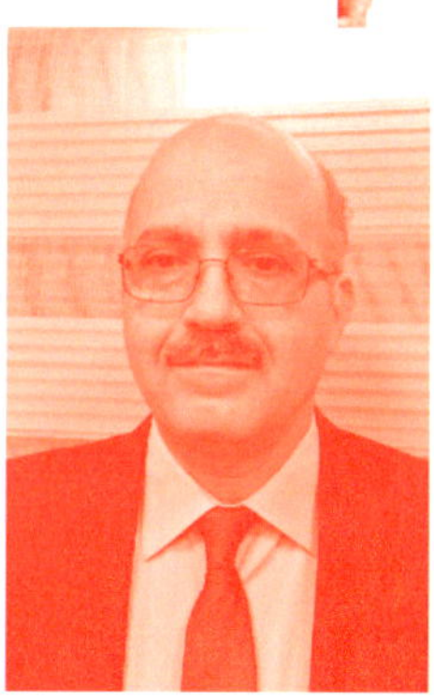
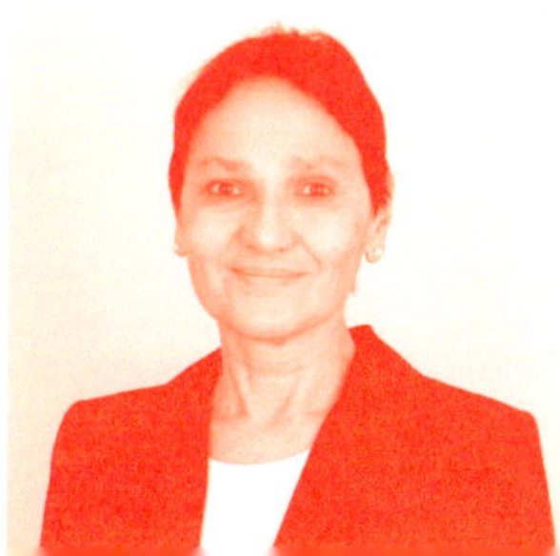
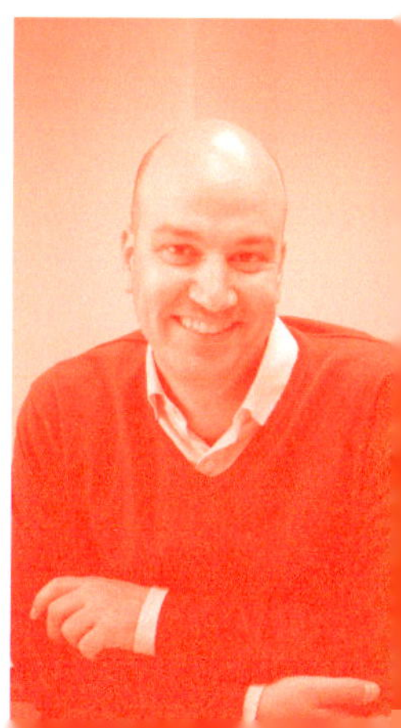

Surgical Challenges in the Management of Liver Disease
http://dx.doi.org/10.5772/intechopen.76553
Edited by Georgios Tsoulfas

Contributors
Carmen Peralta, Maria Eugenia Cornide Petronio, Mónica B. Jiménez-Castro, Esther Bujaldon, Jordi Gracia-Sancho, Julio Cesar Wiederkehr, Barbara Wiederkehr, Henrique Wiederkehr, Ali Ibrahim Yahya, Luis Bredt, Yingzi Ming, Samuel Obiekwe, Georgios Tsoulfas

First published in London, United Kingdom, 2019 by IntechOpen
IntechOpen is the global imprint of INTECHOPEN LIMITED, registered in England and Wales, registration number: 11086078, The Shard, 25th floor, 32 London Bridge Street
London, SE19SG – United Kingdom
Printed in Croatia

British Library Cataloguing-in-Publication Data
A catalogue record for this book is available from the British Library

Additional hard and PDF copies can be obtained from orders@intechopen.com

Surgical Challenges in the Management of Liver Disease
Edited by Georgios Tsoulfas
p. cm.
Print ISBN 978-1-83880-157-1
Online ISBN 978-1-83880-158-8
eBook (PDF) ISBN 978-1-83880-780-1

For EU product safety concerns:
IN TECH d.o.o., Prolaz Marije Krucifikse Kozulić 3, 51000 Rijeka, Croatia, info@intechopen.com or visit our website at intechopen.com.

Meet the editor

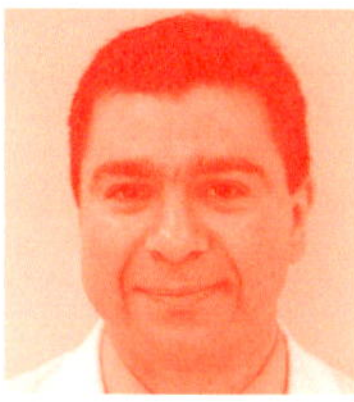

Dr. Georgios Tsoulfas received his medical degree from Brown University School of Medicine and completed his general surgery residency at the University of Iowa Hospitals and Clinics, as well as a transplant research fellowship at the Starzl Transplant Institute at the University of Pittsburgh. He then completed a two-year transplantation surgery fellowship at the Massachusetts General Hospital, Harvard Medical School, and then joined the Division of Solid Organ Transplantation and Hepatobiliary Surgery at the University of Rochester Medical Center as an assistant professor of surgery. He has currently moved back to Greece, where he is an associate professor of surgery at the Aristotle University of Thessaloniki. He has published over 90 papers in peer-reviewed journals and in PubMed, as well as 29 book chapters. He is a reviewer for over 40 international journals and is on the editorial boards of several others.
He is currently the Vice Chair of the International Relations Committee of the American College of Surgeons and the World President of the International College of Surgeons.

Contents

Preface

The complicated nature of hepatic anatomy and physiology, as well as the variety of challenging diseases affecting the liver, have all contributed to the field of hepatic surgery being a highly demanding surgical specialty. The training of a liver surgeon consists of achieving technical expertise, a deep understanding of the intricacies of hepatic anatomy and physiology, experience with acute and chronic liver disease ranging from trauma, infections, benign lesions to primary and metastatic malignancies, as well as knowledge of the continuously evolving technologies. This is necessary to be able to choose correctly from a variety of different treatment methods and different hepatectomy techniques that would be best suited to the specific patient and the specific health problem. The multitude of hepatic surgery techniques involve strategies such as ablation, electroporation, resection with several different instruments, and, last but not least, liver transplantation. At the same time, the physician dealing with these complex issues needs to be aware of the right mix of treatments, as well as the proper sequence. Additionally, it is imperative to possess an understanding of the molecular biology of hepatic function and the evolution of the various diseases to be able to provide patient-targeted therapies.

This book provides an overview of all the above with chapters presenting hepatic anatomy, intricacies of liver physiology as seen in the case of hepatic regeneration and the concept of damage control surgery, challenges and current updates on complex hepatic diseases such as cholangiocarcinoma, and, of course, descriptions of the indications and techniques for some of the more demanding hepatic surgeries such as right hepatectomy and liver transplantation. Its value lies in the fact that the authors present us with their distilled wisdom, which is the result of substantial experience and daily involvement in this most difficult field of medicine and surgery.

Overall, this book should be a useful resource for any physician, whether they are in training or in practice, treating patients with hepatic diseases.

Georgios Tsoulfas, MD, PhD, FICS, FACS,
Associate Professor of Surgery,
Aristotle University of Thessaloniki,
Thessaloniki, Greece

Section 1

Introduction

Chapter 1

Introductory Chapter: Hepatic Surgery

Georgios Tsoulfas

1. Introduction

Hepatic surgery represents one of the more challenging and exciting areas of surgical practice for a variety of reasons. It combines surgical technical expertise with the management of diseases of one of the most vital and elaborate organs of the human organism. Specifically, the liver with its multitude of functions ranging from nutrition, production of energy, clearing and metabolism of a variety of substances and medications, control of the coagulation system, to name a few, represents a human factory with a complex anatomy and physiology. Its various functions make it a central player in a variety of diseases, where irrespective of their benign or malignant nature, can pose significant threats to the whole organism. The main insults faced may include abdominal trauma (with the liver being the second most injured organ), genetic abnormalities, infections, metabolic alterations, and malignancies. The latter can be either primary (hepatocellular carcinoma, cholangiocarcinoma, and hepatoblastoma) or secondary (metastatic hepatic disease from colorectal, neuroendocrine or non-neuroendocrine, and non-colorectal primary). The common feature in all of these diseases is the significant threat that they pose to the human body, as well as the fact that from the multitude of available treatments, surgery is by far the most successful, yet fraught with possible complications and even the possibility of death. This interesting mix allows us to understand the important and challenging nature of hepatic surgery. The liver surgeon needs to possess deep knowledge of hepatic and human physiology, hepatic anatomy, and surgical skill that is a combination of dexterity and patience.

This book with chapters covering the whole spectrum of hepatic surgery represents the cumulative effort of a very experienced group of liver specialists who offer us their distilled experience in areas covering hepatic anatomy with all its significant and often critical variations, an overview of some of the more challenging types of hepatic cancers (such as cholangiocarcinoma), a description of some of the more demanding surgical procedures (such as the extended right hepatectomy), the importance of technology as an extension of the surgeon's eyes and hands (intraoperative hepatic ultrasound), the true meaning of damage control hepatic surgery (typifying the union of understanding hepatic physiology and surgical acumen), and a description of the molecular pathways involved in the evolution and management of liver disease.

The latter carries special weight as we live in the era of precision medicine and patient-targeted treatments. As such, the surgeon should be able to understand the molecular identity of various diseases and how to incorporate that in daily surgical practice. We must learn neither to fear, nor to worship new technology, but rather to objectively and accurately evaluate it and assess its use, and following the appropriate learning curve, incorporate it into our daily practice. The overall goal is to achieve therapy in a safer and more efficient manner for our patients.

Overall, this book represents a true tour de force of a variety of topics having to do with hepatic surgery, as it befits the nature and significance of the subject. It should be stressed that the intended audiences are scientists and physicians and surgeons of different specialties, which all have in common an interest in liver disease and improving the lives of these patients.

Author details

Georgios Tsoulfas
Aristotle University of Thessaloniki, Thessaloniki, Greece

*Address all correspondence to: tsoulfasg@gmail.com

Section 2

Basic Principles in Hepatic Surgery

Chapter 2

Hepatic Regeneration Under Warm or Cold Ischemia Conditions: Controversies and New Approaches

Maria Eugenia Cornide-Petronio, Mónica B. Jiménez-Castro, Esther Bujaldon, Jordi Gracia-Sancho and Carmen Peralta

Abstract

Ischemia-reperfusion (I/R) associated with hepatic resection and living related liver transplantation is an unsolved problem in clinical practice. Indeed, I/R induces damage and regenerative failure in clinical liver surgery. Signaling pathways regarding the pathophysiology of liver I/R and regeneration making clear distinction between situations of cold and warm ischemia, as well as liver regeneration with or without vascular occlusion, will be addressed. The different experimental models used to date to improve the postoperative outcomes in clinical liver surgery will be also described. Furthermore, the most updated therapeutic strategies, as well as the clinical and scientific controversies in the field, will be discussed. Such information may be useful to guide the design of better experimental models as well as the effective therapeutic strategies in liver surgery that can succeed in achieving its clinical application.

Keywords: liver surgery, regeneration, ischemia–reperfusion injury, warm ischemia, cold ischemia

1. Introduction

Any surgical situation involving liver hepatectomy requires subsequent regeneration in order to restore the liver/body ratio. The liver's ability to restore tissue after loss depends on the interaction of numerous cells and a complex network of mediators [1]. In most cases, in clinical practice, liver surgery involves both ischemia-reperfusion (I/R) injury and regeneration [1]. Liver I/R injury is a pathophysiological event that occurs during surgical interventions such as liver resection or liver transplantation (LT); it controls bleeding during parenchymal dissection and has a significant effect on liver function prognosis [2–6]. I/R injury is a two-stage phenomenon in which cell damage due to hypoxia and the lack of biomechanical stimulus is exacerbated upon the restoration of oxygen delivery and shear stress [7]. However, I/R injury is inevitable in liver surgery and significantly reduces the organ's regeneration after hepatectomy [1]. Mechanisms of liver I/R injury are complex; they include mainly microcirculation failure and the related oxidative stress, a series of cellular and molecular responses, and the interaction between hepatocytes, liver sinusoidal endothelial cells, hepatic stellate cells, Kupffer cells, infiltrating neutrophils, macrophages, and platelets [2, 7–11].

Liver I/R injury involves great many factors and mediators. The associations between the signaling pathways are extremely complex, and at present, the events occurring between the start of reperfusion and the final outcome (either poor function or a nonfunctional liver graft) are not fully understood [6]. The extent and timing of ischemia, the type of liver undergoing I/R, and the existence of liver regeneration may alter the mechanisms of liver I/R injury and the effects of the treatment strategies assessed to date [12]. This point was exemplified by Ramalho et al. who demonstrated the loss of protection against liver damage of Ang-II receptor antagonists in conditions of partial hepatectomy (PH), while in conditions of I/R without hepatectomy, the Ang-II receptor antagonists decreased liver damage [13]. As is well known, the mechanisms of liver damage differ according to the percentage of the liver mass deprived of blood [14]. Therefore, experimental models that reproduce as closely as possible the clinical conditions in which these strategies are applied are likely to lead to the implementation of strategies in clinical practice in the relatively short term [1].

In this chapter, we aim to show that the mechanisms that govern liver I/R injury and regeneration depend on the experimental model applied. These models are valuable tools for elucidating the physiopathology of liver I/R injury and uncovering new therapeutic targets and drugs. A number of strategies for protecting the liver from I/R injury and for improving liver regeneration have been developed in animal models, some of which may find their way into clinical practice [6]. We stress that the type of ischemia (cold or warm) has an important influence in liver surgery, but most of the currently available reviews on the mechanisms of I/R do not distinguish between them [6]. In our view, this information may help to guide the design of future experimental models and treatment strategies in liver surgery for use in clinical practice.

2. Hepatic regeneration under warm ischemia

Following PH, hepatocytes that are normally quiescent enter the cell cycle in order to replace the part that has been removed. The original liver mass is restored after some 6–8 weeks (in humans) by tightly synchronized rounds of replication of the remaining hepatocytes [15]. Self-replication of the existing individual cell types is thought to be the key mechanism of regeneration after PH. However, it was recently suggested that hepatic progenitor cells may contribute to liver regeneration following PH [15]. A vast number of growth and metabolic factors and cytokines simultaneously regulate liver regeneration during PH. Under the influence of innate immunity components and gut-derived lipopolysaccharide, on Kupffer cells and stellate cells, tumor necrosis factor alpha, and interleukin 6, provided by those cells, prepares hepatocytes to respond to growth factors like epidermal growth factor and hepatocyte growth factor [15]. Among other auxiliary mitogens are norepinephrine, Notch and jagged proteins, vascular endothelial growth factor, platelet-derived growth factor, bile acids, insulin serotonin, estrogens leptin, triodothronine, and FGF1 and 2 [16]. Joint signals from these factors lead to the progression of the liver cell cycle, which in turn results in DNA synthesis and ultimately the proliferation of liver cells as mentioned above [15].

As is well known, remnant liver following PH can be used as an in vivo liver regeneration model in order to assess possible treatment strategies for improving postoperative outcomes after hepatectomy. Nonetheless, a two-third partial hepatectomy alone does not cause death in these models, and the remnant liver has the capacity to regenerate. In contrast, 30 min of liver ischemia just before PH exacerbates the remnant liver function, causing high mortality and negatively affecting liver weight restoration [1, 17]. It is also well known that vascular occlusion of the hepatic hilum is often used to avoid hemorrhage in liver resection. However, vascular occlusion has been associated with warm ischemia damage, resulting in significant organ dysfunction and regenerative failure [12]. Hepatocytes are severely affected by I/R, especially in normothermic ischemia. Most of the early changes in anoxic hepatocytes take place in the mitochondria. Briefly, due to the unavailability of O_2 as a terminal electron carrier for the mitochondrial respiratory chain, the electron flow is immediately interrupted, thus reducing the respiratory chain. Since the mitochondria no longer accept electrons from substrates, pyridine nucleotides decrease, thus causing a rise in the intracellular $NADH/NAD^+$ ratio. The disruption of oxidative phosphorylation rapidly depletes cellular ATP, accelerates glycolysis, increases lactate formation, and alters H^+, Na^+, and Ca^{2+} homeostasis and thus induces severe damage to the hepatocyte. Ischemia also causes a substantial rise in cAMP, a key factor in glucose metabolism. Via the action of cAMP-dependent protein kinase, cAMP causes the phosphorylation/deregulation of enzymes, which play a major role in the control of carbohydrate metabolism [18, 19]. Reperfusion injury derives mainly from toxic reactive oxygen species (ROS) generated on the reintroduction of O_2 to ischemic tissues. ROS are produced both from intracellular and from extracellular sources; in liver cells, the mitochondria are their major source [7, 20].

3. Preclinical studies in normothermic hepatic ischemia associated with hepatic resection

3.1 Animal species used

The results of animal studies can be extrapolated to human beings, even though there are limitations such as the differences in ischemia tolerance, the anatomy of the organ in different species, and differences in the surgical conditions applied in clinical practice and in experimental models [21]. Therefore, the correct choice of animal species and experimental model, and the standardization of the protocol according to the clinical issue under study, is particularly important [14]. Small animals like rats and mice are exceptionally useful because they are easy to handle, present minimal, financial, logistical or ethical problems, and allow genetic alterations such as the creation of transgenic and knock-out animals [14]. Larger animals (pigs, sheep, and dogs) have a more similar anatomy and physiology to humans, but their use is restricted by serious financial and logistical difficulties, ethical concerns, and the limited availability of immunological tools for use in these species [14, 21]. The age and sex of animals are also issues to consider. With regard to age, there are significant differences between younger (35–50 g) and older rats (250–400 g) in terms of their hepatic microcirculation at the different stages of ischemia, and with regard to sex, female rats are more sensitive to reperfusion injury than males after normothermic ischemia [14, 22, 23].

3.2 Experimental models of normothermic hepatic ischemia to evaluate the mechanisms involved

3.2.1 Global hepatic ischemia with portocaval decompression

The Pringle maneuver is often applied during liver resection, due to safety concerns. However, it has been associated with delayed liver failure and poor prognosis in patients undergoing major hepatectomy in conditions of prolonged liver ischemia [1, 13]. The global liver ischemia model with portal decompression provides an ideal simulation of the clinical condition of warm ischemia after the Pringle maneuver for liver resection and transplant [6, 14]. The first successful shunt operation carried out in humans was by Vidal in 1903 [24]. Blakemore was among the first researchers to report successful portal-systemic anastomosis in rats, working mainly with endothelium-lined tubes [25]. Burnett et al. modified the technique to create a portocaval shunt [26]. In 1959, Bernstein and Cheiker developed the portosystemic shunt, which led portal blood into one of the iliac veins after functional hepatectomy [27]. In small animals, many other shunt techniques have been developed such as the portofemoral shunt or the mesentericocaval shunt via the jugular vein. In 1995, the splenocaval shunt was developed by Spiegel [28]. In large animals, on the other hand, a porto-femoro jugular bypass is frequently used [14, 29]. Results from experimental models of hepatic I/R injury alone are often extrapolated to clinical liver resection with PH and ischemia. However, in conventional experimental I/R models (for example, 70% partial hepatic ischemia), reperfusion ensues in the presence of nonischemic lobes [1]. Experimental models that combine PH and I/R injury rule out any contribution to recovery of the nonaffected liver tissue. Furthermore, in this model, postischemic recovery depends on the liver cell damage caused by the IR-injury and also on the stress caused by the liver resection and posthepatectomy liver regeneration [1, 30].

3.2.2 Global liver ischemia with spleen transposition

In 1970, Bengmark et al. developed this model for surgical treatment of portal hypertension [31]. In 1981, Meredith and Wade described a rat model that produced a portosystemic shunt in the anhepatic rat by transposition of the spleen, making a small incision in the left hypochondrium [32]. With the spleen inside a subcutaneous pouch, adequate portosystemic anastomoses emerge after some 2–3 weeks. The transposition induces the reversal of the blood flow in the splenic vein, which stimulates angiogenesis. Two weeks later, in the second step, a median laparotomy and temporary occlusion of the hepatoduodenal ligament are performed. This decompression by spleen transposition is easy to perform, because it does not require microsurgery. Within 2 or 3 weeks of surgery, the spleen is encapsulated without any signs of inflammation or bleeding. One drawback of this model is the long time span (3 weeks) until adequate portosystemic collaterals are large enough to take full control of portal vein flow. Furthermore, the effect of the changes in hepatic inflow on the collaterals remains unclear [6, 14, 33].

3.2.3 Partial hepatic resection under vascular occlusion

In 1982, Yamauchi et al. reported a hepatic ischemia model in which ischemia is induced by occlusion of the hepatic artery, the portal vein, and the bile duct of the left and median lobes. No extracorporeal shunt is required because the blood continues to flow through the right and caudal liver lobes. This model of partial ischemia (70%) has been extensively used in experimental studies of hepatic I/R [34–36]. An experimental model of 30% partial liver ischemia has also been used, in which occlusion at the hepatic artery and portal vein interrupts the supply of blood to the right lobe of the liver [19]. In the clinical setting, PH under I/R is normally performed to control bleeding during parenchymal dissection [6]. Therefore, an experimental model incorporating both hepatic regeneration and I/R injury can simulate the clinical situation of selective or hemihepatic vascular occlusion for liver resections. In this model, after left hepatic lobe resection, a microvascular clamp is placed across the portal triad supplying the median lobe (30%). Congestion of the bowel is prevented during the clamping because the portal flow through the right and caudate lobes is preserved. At the end of ischemia, the right lobe and caudate lobes are resected, and the clamp is released to achieve reperfusion of the median lobe. In this hepatic resection model, portal decompression is not required, and certain important criteria are also met, such as reversibility, good reproducibility, and ease of execution [14, 19, 37].

3.3 Strategies applied in experimental models of normothermic ischemia

Many experimental studies have set out to develop in vivo pharmacological strategies for inhibiting the harmful effects of warm I/R [38–46]. Some of these studies are summarized in **Table 1**. However, none of them have been able to prevent hepatic I/R injury [6, 14]. However, it is important to develop strategies in experimental models that reproduce clinical practice conditions as closely as possible: for example, the use of intermittent clamping, and the combination of PH and I/R injury. Few of the studies carried out to date have complied with these requirements [12]. Some of these studies are summarized in **Table 2**. Recent breakthroughs in molecular biology are providing new opportunities for applying gene therapy to reduce liver I/R injury. The experimental data, however, have highlighted several problems inherent in gene therapy, including vector toxicity, difficulties in increasing transfection efficiency and protein expression at the appropriate site and time, and the difficulty of obtaining adequate mutants.

	Warm ischemia	
	Mice	
Drug	**Ischemic time**	**Effect**
Cerulenin	15 min	↓ UPC2, ↑ ATP
Platinum nanoparticles		↓ Hepatic injury
Exendin 4	20 min	↓ Hepatic injury and autophagy
Catalase and derivatives	30 min	↓ Oxidative stress
Apocynin		↓ Oxidative stress
Allopurinol		↓ Oxidative stress
N-Acetylcysteine	40, 90 min	↓ Hepatic injury, oxidative stress and apoptosis
Dipyridamole	45 min	↓ Hepatic injury
15-deoxy-$\Delta^{12,14}$-prostaglandin J_2	60 min	↓ Hepatic injury and inflammation
Ago-miR-46a		↓ Hepatic injury and apoptosis
Cold-inducible RNA-binding protein (CIRP) blockade		↓ Hepatic injury, apoptosis and inflammation
Anti-CD25 antibody		↓ Hepatic injury and inflammation
Diannexin		↓ Hepatic injury and inflammation
Ethyl pyruvate		↓ Hepatic injury, apoptosis and autophagy
Fasting		↓ Hepatic injury and inflammation; ↑ autophagy
Angiotensin II receptor antagonist		↓ Hepatic injury, apoptosis and inflammation
Riboflavin		↓ Hepatic injury, oxidative stress and inflammation
α7 Nicotinic acetylcholine receptor agonist		↓ Hepatic injury, oxidative stress and inflammation
Omega–3 Fatty acid		↓ Hepatic injury and inflammation; ↑ liver regeneration
Cobalt protoporphyrin	60, 90 min	↓ Hepatic injury and inflammation

Warm ischemia		
Mice		
Drug	**Ischemic time**	**Effect**
Hydroxytyrosol	75 min	↓ Hepatic injury, apoptosis, oxidative stress and inflammation
miR-370 inhibitor		↓ Hepatic injury and inflammation
Augmenter of liver regeneration (ALR)	90 min	↓ Hepatic injury, apoptosis and inflammation
Carbon monoxide		↓ Hepatic injury
Pan-selectin antagonist		↓ Inflammation
Erythropoietin		↓ Hepatic injury and apoptosis
Helium		↓ Hepatic injury; ↑ survival
Low-dose LPS		↓ Hepatic injury, apoptosis and inflammation
Protease-activated receptor 4 antagonist		↓ Hepatic injury, apoptosis and inflammation
Vasoactive intestinal peptide neuropeptide		↓ Hepatic injury, apoptosis and inflammation
Rats		
Drug	**Ischemic time**	**Effect**
ACE inhibitor	30 min	↓ Oxidative stress
ROS scavenger		↓ Apoptosis
Branched-chain amino acid (BCAA)		↓ Hepatic injury and inflammation
Carvacrol		↓ Hepatic injury, apoptosis and oxidative stress
CR2-CD59 (complement inhibitor)		↓ Hepatic injury; ↑ regeneration and survival
Hydrolysed whey peptide		↓ Hepatic injury, apoptosis and inflammation
Hyperbaric oxygen therapy		↓ Hepatic injury
Sivelestat sodium hydrate		↓ Hepatic injury and inflammation
Liraglutide		↓ Hepatic injury, apoptosis and inflammation
Allopurinol	30, 60 min	↓Oxidative stress
Diazoxide		↓ Hepatic injury and inflammation
PPARα agonist	30, 60, 90 min	↓ Oxidative stress and inflammation; ↑ autophagy
Propofol73		↓ Hepatic injury and apoptosis
Melatonin	35, 40 min	↓ Hepatic injury, apoptosis and oxidative stress
Levosimendan	40, 60 min	↓ Hepatic injury, apoptosis, oxidative stress and inflammation
Carnosic acid	45 min	↓ Hepatic injury
Limonin		↓ Hepatic injury, oxidative stress and inflammation
Low-intensity laser therapy		↓ Hepatic injury and oxidative stress
Rho-kinase inhibitor		↓ Hepatic injury; ↑ survival
Cardamonin		↓ Hepatic injury, oxidative stress and inflammation
Quercetin		↓ Hepatic Injury
Protoporphyrin		↓ Hepatic Injury

SOD	45, 60 min	↓ Inflammation
L-arginine		↓ Inflammation
Tocopherol	45, 90 min	↓ Oxidative stress and inflammation
IL-10	60 min	↓ Oxidative stress and inflammation
Anti-ICAM-1		↓ Inflammation
Gabexate mesilate		↓ Inflammation
Analogue of prostacyclin (OP-2507)		↓ Inflammation
n-3 PUFA		↓ Hepatic injury and oxidative stress
Adiponectin		↓ Hepatic injury, apoptosis and inflammation
Atorvastatin		↓ Hepatic injury and inflammation
Dexmedetomidine		↓ Hepatic injury and oxidative stress
Dioscin		↓ Hepatic injury, apoptosis and inflammation
Fibrin-derived peptide Bβ15–42		↓ Hepatic injury and inflammation
L-α-glycerylphosphorylcholine (GPC)		↓ Hepatic injury and oxidative stress
Rapamycin		↓ Hepatic injury; ↑ autophagy
Rosmarinic acid		↓ Hepatic injury, oxidative stress and inflammation
Sevoflurane		↓ Hepatic injury and oxidative stress
Simvastatin		↓ Hepatic injury, apoptosis and inflammation
Crocin		↓ Hepatic injury and oxidative stress
Tert-butylhydroquinone		↓ Inflammation
Hydrogen-rich saline		↓ Hepatic injury and oxidative stress
Spermine NONOate	60, 90 min	↓ Oxidative stress and inflammation
FK506		↓ Inflammation
Chloroquine		↓ Hepatic injury and inflammation
Lithium		↓ Hepatic injury and inflammation
AMPK activators	90 min	↑ NO, ATP
α-Lipoic acid		↓ Apoptosis; ↑ liver regeneration
Edaravone		↓ Hepatic injury and oxidative stress
Reduced glutathione		↓ Hepatic injury, apoptosis and oxidative stress
Sildenafil		↓ Hepatic injury, apoptosis and inflammation
Oleanolic		↓ Hepatic injury; ↑ survival
Unacylated-ghrelin		↓ Oxidative stress
Minocycline	2, 6 and 24 h	↓ Hepatic injury, oxidative stress and inflammation
	Pigs	
Drug	**Ischemic time**	**Effect**
Sevoflurane	40 min	↓ Hepatic injury

Table 1.
Pharmacological strategies used in experimental models of warm ischemia.

Warm ischemia with partial hepatectomy		
Mice		
Drug	**Ischemic time**	**Effect**
Low dose of 2-complement receptor 1-related protein Y	30 min	↓ Hepatic injury and oxidative stress; ↑ liver regeneration
Melatonin	60 min	↓ Hepatic injury; ↑ liver regeneration
C1 esterase inhibitor		↓ Hepatic injury; ↑ liver regeneration and survival
Hydrogen sulfide	75, 90 min	↓ Hepatic injury and apoptosis; ↑ survival and liver regeneration
Rats		
Drug	**Ischemic time**	**Effect**
CF102	10 min	↓ Hepatic injury, apoptosis and inflammation; ↑ liver regeneration
Inchinkoto	15, 30 min	↓ Hepatic injury, oxidative stress and inflammation
Anti-HMGB1	20 min	↓ Hepatic injury; ↑ liver regeneration
Thrombomodulin		↓ Hepatic injury and apoptosis; ↑ liver regeneration
2mercaptoethane sulfonate	30 min	↓ Hepatic injury and oxidative stress; ↑ liver regeneration
Butyrate	30, 60 min	↓ Hepatic injury and inflammation
Omega3 fatty acids	40 min	↓ Hepatic injury and oxidative stress
Polyamines		↓ Necrosis, apoptosis and inflammation; ↑ liver regeneration
Glucose or lipid emulsion	60 min	↓ Hepatic injury; ↑ liver regeneration
Resistin or anti-visfatin antibodies		↓ Hepatic injury; ↑ liver regeneration
Tauroursodeoxycholate		↓ Oxidative stress
Sirolimus		↓ Inflammation
Combined angiotensin II receptor type 1 and 2 antagonists		↓ Hepatic injury and oxidative stress; ↑ liver regeneration
Thymoquinone		↓ Hepatic injury, apoptosis and oxidative stress
M3 AChR antagonist		↓ Hepatic injury and inflammation; ↑ regeneration and survival
Hydrogen sulfide	75, 90 min	↓ Hepatic injury, apoptosis and inflammation; ↑ regeneration and survival
IL-1 receptor antagonist	90 min	↓ Oxidative stress
Pigs		
Drug	**Ischemic time**	**Effect**
Hydrogen inhalation	20 min	↓ Hepatic injury, apoptosis and oxidative stress
Desferrioxamine	150 min	↓ Oxidative stress; ↑ liver function
Dogs		
Drug	**Ischemic time**	**Effect**
FK 3311 (Cox-2 inhibitor)	60 min	↓ Inflammation

Table 2.
Pharmacological strategies used in experimental models of warm ischemia with partial hepatectomy.

4. Controversies on hepatic regeneration under warm or cold ischemia

In an attempt to expand the size of the donor pool, the use of living related liver transplantation (LDLT) has helped increase the number of donor livers, but, nonetheless, concerns persist about graft-size disparity and hepatic regeneration. In 1990, Broelsch et al. reported the first 20 series of LDLT in the USA [47]. In 1997, Lo et al. [48] performed the first successful LDLT using an extended right lobe from a living donor for an adult recipient [6]. In LDLT, liver graft must be successfully regenerated; however, cold I/R, which will take place during liver transplantation surgery, will reduce the regenerative capacity of the liver.

The clinical application of strategies designed at beachside will depend on the use of experimental models that resemble as much as possible the clinical conditions in which the strategy intends to be applied [12]. However, many investigators have used rodent models of PH under or without vascular occlusion to mimic some of the pathophysiological events that occur during LT [6]. To the best of our knowledge, pharmacological strategies, which were used in experimental models of hepatic regeneration under warm ischemia (**Table 2**), were not applied in experimental models of LDLT. However, only three drugs (sirolimus, Ang II receptor type 2 antagonist, and Omega-3) were applied in patients submitted to LDLT (see **Table 3**). In contrast with the benefits on liver regeneration observed in experimental models of PH under I/R [49], the administration of sirolimus in LDLT decreases liver regeneration in patients [50]. Indeed, sirolimus decreases liver injury in patients only in combination with cyclosporine [51]. Similarly, angiotensin II receptor type 2 antagonist does not reduce hepatic injury as opposed to the benefits obtained in preclinical studies of PH under vascular occlusion [13, 52]. By contrast, pharmacological treatment with omega-3 had benefits on hepatic injury in clinical LDLT and in preclinical studies after PH under vascular occlusion [53, 54]. In our view, these controversial results may be explained at least partially, by the differences in the mechanism responsible of I/R damage and liver regenerative failure dependently on the surgical procedure (LDLT versus PH + I/R). Of note, it would be extremely useful to make a clear distinction between the mechanisms for each surgical situation to design therapies that demonstrate its effectiveness under experimental conditions similar to what happens in clinical practice [12]. This will probably lead to translation of the best strategies to clinical practice in the short term [12].

Living donor liver transplantation		
Human		
Drug	**Ischemic time**	**Effect**
Sirolimus	Not reported	↓ Liver regeneration
Sirolimus + cyclosporine		↓ Hepatic injury
Angiotensin II receptor type 2 antagonist		↑ Hepatic injury
Omega3		↓ Hepatic injury; ↑ liver regeneration

Table 3.
Pharmacological strategies used in living donor liver transplantation.

5. Conclusions

Although our knowledge about the mechanisms involved in the development of liver I/R injury and regenerative failure has significantly improved, and it has consequently been accompanied by a long list of potential therapeutic alternatives, I/R injury and regenerative failure after surgical procedure still represent a serious problem in the clinical practice. It should be considered that the mechanisms involved in hepatic I/R and regenerative failure very much depend on the experimental conditions used: which type of research is done, type of ischemia applied (warm or cold), period of ischemia (ranging from minutes to days), extension of hepatic ischemia (partial or total), graft subclinical situation (healthy, steatotic, aged,...), etc. Thus, new therapeutic strategies from experimental studies should be considered specific to the concrete experimental/surgical conditions used, and most probably, they cannot automatically be validated for all clinical situations requiring both vascular occlusion and liver regeneration [7]. We recognize the complication, but multidisciplinary research groups should devote additional efforts to better understand the cellular alterations and the crosstalk within the liver during the different clinical setting, requiring both vascular occlusion and liver regeneration to ultimately develop effectual therapeutic strategies aimed at reducing I/R damage and improving hepatic regeneration after liver surgery.

Acknowledgements

This research was supported by the Ministerio de Economía y Competitividad (project grant SAF-2015-64857-R) Madrid, Spain; the European Union (FondosFeder, “una manera de hacer Europa”); by CERCA Program/Generalitat de Catalunya; and by the Secretaria d’Universitats i Recerca (Grant 2017SGR-551) Barcelona, Spain. ME Cornide-Petronio has a Sara Borrell contract from the Instituto de Salud Carlos III (Grant CD15/00129), Madrid, Spain. MB Jiménez-Castro has a contract from the Programa de Promoción del talento y su empleabilidad from the Ministerio de Economía y Competitividad (Grant EMP-TU-2015-4167), Madrid, Spain. J Gracia-Sancho received continuous funding from the Instituto de Salud Carlos III (currently FIS PI17/00012) & the CIBEREHD, from Ministerio de Ciencia, Innovación y Universidades.

Conflict of interest

The authors declare that they have no conflict of interest.

Author details

Maria Eugenia Cornide-Petronio[1†], Mónica B. Jiménez-Castro[2†], Esther Bujaldon[1], Jordi Gracia-Sancho[3] and Carmen Peralta[1,4,5]*

1 Institut d'Investigacions Biomèdiques August Pi i Sunyer (IDIBAPS), Barcelona, Spain

2 Transplant Biomedicals, S.L., Barcelona, Spain

3 Barcelona Hepatic Hemodynamic Laboratory, Institut d'Investigacions Biomèdiques August Pi i Sunyer (IDIBAPS), Hospital Clínic de Barcelona, Centro de Investigaciones Biomédicas en Red en Enfermedades Hepáticas y Digestivas (CIBEREHD), Barcelona, Spain

4 Centro de Investigación Biomédica en Red de Enfermedades Hepáticas y Digestivas (CIBEREHD), Barcelona, Spain

5 Facultad de Medicina, Universidad International de Cataluña, Barcelona, Spain

*Address all correspondence to: cperalta@clinic.ub.es

† Both authors contributed equally to this work.

References

[1] Casillas-Ramirez A, Escobedo-Medina SG, Cordero-Pérez P, Jiménez-Castro MB, Peralta C. Ischemia-reperfusion injury and oxidative stress. In: Gracia, Salvado, editors. Gastrointestinal Tissue: Oxidative Stress and Dietary Antioxidants. London: Elsevier INC; 2016. pp. 141-154

[2] Fu P, Li W. Nitric oxide in liver ischemia-reperfusion injury. In: Muriel P, editor. Liver Pathophysiology. London: Elsevier INC; 2017. pp. 125-127

[3] Clavien P, Harvey P, Strasberg S. Preservation and reperfusion injuries in liver allografts. An overview and synthesis of current studies. Transplantation. 1992;**53**:957-978

[4] Huguet C, Gavelli A, Chieco P, Bona S, Harb J, Joseph J, et al. Liver ischemia for hepatic resection: Where is the limit? Surgery. 1992;**111**:251-259

[5] Serafin A, Rosello-Catafau J, Prats N, Xaus C, Gelpi E, Peralta C. Ischemic preconditioning increases the tolerance of fatty liver to hepatic ischemia-reperfusion injury in the rat. The American Journal of Pathology. 2002;**161**:587-601. DOI: 10.1016/S0002-9440(10)64214-9

[6] Jiménez-Castro MB, Elias-Miró M, Casillas-Ramirez A, Peralta C. Experimental models in liver surgery. In: Abdeldayem, editor. Hepatic Surgery. Rijeka: InTech Open; 2013. pp. 121-166

[7] Peralta C, Jiménez-Castro MB, Gracia-Sancho J. Hepatic ischemia and reperfusion injury: Effects on the liver sinusoidal milieu. Journal of Hepatology. 2013;**59**:1094-1106. DOI: 10.1016/j.jhep.2013.06.017

[8] Selzner N, Rudiger H, Graf R, Clavien P. Protective strategies against ischemic injury of the liver. Gastroenterology. 2003;**125**:917-936

[9] Jaeschke H. Molecular mechanisms of hepatic ischemia-reperfusion injury and preconditioning. American Journal of Physiology. Gastrointestinal and Liver Physiology. 2003;**284**:G15-G26. DOI: 10.1152/ajpgi.00342.2002

[10] Montalvo-Jave EE, Escalante-Tattersfield T, Ortega-Salgado JA, Piña E, Geller DA. Factors in the pathophysiology of the liver ischemia-reperfusion injury. The Journal of Surgical Research. 2008;**147**:153-159. DOI: 10.1016/j.jss.2007.06.015

[11] Gracia-Sancho J, Villarreal G Jr, Zhang Y, Yu JX, Liu Y, Tullius SG, et al. Flow cessation triggers endothelial dysfunction during organ cold storage conditions: Strategies for pharmacologic intervention. Transplantation. 2010;**90**:142-149. DOI: 10.1097/TP.0b013e3181e228db

[12] Gracia-Sancho J, Casillas-Ramírez A, Peralta C. Molecular pathways in protecting the liver from ischaemia/reperfusion injury: A 2015 update. Clinical Science (London, England). 2015;**129**:345-362. DOI: 10.1042/CS20150223

[13] Ramalho FS, Alfany-Fernandez I, Casillas-Ramirez A, Massip-Salcedo M, Serafín A, Rimola A, Arroyo V, Rodés J, Roselló-Catafau J, Peralta C. Are angiotensin II receptor antagonists useful strategies in steatotic and nonsteatotic livers in conditions of partial hepatectomy under ischemia-reperfusion? The Journal of Pharmacology and Experimental Therapeutics. 2009;**329**:130-140. DOI: 10.1124/jpet.108.147835

[14] Mendes-Braz M, Elias-Miró M, Jiménez-Castro MB, Casillas-Ramírez A, Ramalho FS, Peralta C. The current state of knowledge of

hepatic ischemia-reperfusion injury based on its study in experimental models. Journal of Biomedicine & Biotechnology. 2012;**2012**:298657. DOI: 10.1155/2012/298657

[15] Katoonizadeh A. Liver Regeneration. In: Muriel P, editor. Liver Pathophysiology. London: Elsevier INC; 2017. pp. 113-123

[16] Mao SA, Glorioso JM, Nyberg SL. Liver regeneration. Translational Research. 2014;**163**:352-362. DOI: 10.1016/j.trsl.2014.01.005

[17] Ito K, Ozasa H, Horikawa S. Effects of prior splenectomy on remnant liver after partial hepatectomy with Pringle maneuver in rats. Liver International. 2005;**25**:438-444. DOI: 10.1111/j.1478-3231.2005.01102.x

[18] Gasbarrini A, Borle AB, Farghali H, Bender C, Francavilla A, Van Thiel D. Effect of anoxia on intracellular ATP, Na+i, Ca2+i, Mg2+i, and cytotoxicity in rat hepatocytes. The Journal of Biological Chemistry. 1992;**267**:6654-6663

[19] Peralta C, Bartrons R, Riera L, Manzano A, Xaus C, Gelpí E, Roselló-Catafau J. Hepatic preconditioning preserves energy metabolism during sustained ischemia. American Journal of Physiology. Gastrointestinal and Liver Physiology. 2000;**279**:G163-G171. DOI: 10.1152/ajpgi.2000.279.1.G163

[20] Caraceni P, Domenicali M, Vendemiale G, Grattagliano I, Pertosa A, Nardo B, et al. The reduced tolerance of rat fatty liver to ischemia reperfusion is associated with mitochondrial oxidative injury. The Journal of Surgical Research. 2005;**124**:160-168. DOI: 10.1016/j.jss.2004.10.007

[21] Cornide-Petronio ME, Casillas-Ramirez A, Jiménez-Castro MB, Peralta C. Experimental brain death models in liver transplantation. In: Tsoulfas, editor. Organ Donation and Transplantation. London: InTechOpen; 2018. pp. 135-151

[22] Yahanda A, Paidas C, Clemens M. Susceptibility of hepatic microcirculation to reperfusion injury: A comparison of adult and suckling rats. Journal of Pediatric Surgery. 1990;**25**:208-213

[23] Gasbarrini A, Addolorato G, Di Campli C, Simoncini M, Montemagn M, Castagneto M, et al. Gender affects reperfusion injury in rat liver. Digestive Diseases and Sciences. 2001;**46**:1305-1312

[24] Vidal M. Traitement chirurgical des ascites. La Presse Médicale. 1903;**11**:747-749

[25] Blakemore A, Lord J. The technic of using vitallium tubes in establishing portacaval shunts for portal hypertension. Annals of Surgery. 1945;**122**:449-475

[26] Burnett W, Rosemond G, Weston J, Tyson R. Studies of hepatic response to changes in blood supply. Surgical Forum. 1951;**94**:147-153

[27] Bernstein D, Cheiker S. Simple technique for Porto-caval shunt in the rat. Journal of Applied Physiology. 1959;**14**:467-470

[28] Spiegel H, Bremer C, Boin C, Langer M. Reduction of hepatic injury by indomethacin-mediated vasoconstriction: A rat model with temporary splenocaval shunt. Journal of Investigative Surgery. 1995;**8**:363-369

[29] Uhlmann D, Armann B, Gaebel G, Ludwig S, Hess J, Pietsch U, et al. Endothelin A receptor blockade reduces hepatic ischemia/reperfusion injury after warm ischemia in a pig model. Journal of Gastrointestinal Surgery. 2003;**7**:331-339

[30] He S, Atkinson C, Qiao F, Cianflone K, Chen X, Tomlinson S. A complement-dependent balance between hepatic ischemia/reperfusion injury and liver regeneration in mice. The Journal of Clinical Investigation. 2009;**119**:2304-2316. DOI: 10.1172/JCI38289

[31] Bengmark S, Börjesson B, Olin T, Sakuma S, Vosmic J. Subcutaneous transposition of the spleen: An experimental study in the rat. Scandinavian Journal of Gastroenterology. Supplement. 1970;**7**:175-179

[32] Meredith C, Wade D. A model of portal-systemic shunting in the rat. Clinical and Experimental Pharmacology & Physiology. 1981;**8**:651-652

[33] Suzuki S, Nakamura S, Sakaguchi T, Mitsuoka H, Tsuchiya Y, Kojima Y, et al. Pathophysiological appraisal of a rat model of total hepatic ischemia with an extracorporeal portosystemic shunt. The Journal of Surgical Research. 1998;**80**(1):22-27. DOI: 10.1006/jsre.1998.5419

[34] Hasselgren P, Jennische E, Fornander J, Hellman A. No beneficial affect of ATP-MgCl2 on impaired transmembrane potential and protein synthesis in liver ischemia. Acta Chirurgica Scandinavica. 1982;**148**:601-607

[35] Massip-Salcedo M, Zaouali M, Padrissa-Altés S, Casillas-Ramírez A, Rodés J, Roselló-Catafau J, Peralta C. Activation of peroxisome proliferator-activated receptor-alpha inhibits the injurious effects of adiponectin in rat steatotic liver undergoing ischemia-reperfusion. Hepatology. 2008;**47**:461-472. DOI: 10.1002/hep.21935

[36] Casillas-Ramírez A, Amine-Zaouali M, Massip-Salcedo M, Padrissa-Altés S, Bintanel-Morcillo M, Ramalho F, et al. Inhibition of angiotensin II action protects rat steatotic livers against ischemia-reperfusion injury. Critical Care Medicine. 2008;**36**:1256-1266. DOI: 10.1097/CCM.0b013e31816a023c

[37] Palmes D, Spiegel H. Animal models of liver regeneration. Biomaterials. 2004;**25**:1601-1611

[38] Elias-Miro M, Massip-Salcedo M, Jiménez-Castro MB, Peralta C. Does adiponectin benefit steatotic liver transplantation? Liver Transplantation. 2011;**17**:993-1004. DOI: 10.1002/lt.22358

[39] Fernández L, Heredia N, Grande L, Gómez G, Rimola A, Marco A, et al. Preconditioning protects liver and lung damage in rat liver transplantation: Role of xanthine/xanthine oxidase. Hepatology. 2002;**36**:562-572. DOI: 10.1053/jhep.2002.34616

[40] Serafin A, Rosello-Catafau J, Prats N, Gelpi E, Rodes J, Peralta C. Ischemic preconditioning affects interleukin release in fatty livers of rats undergoing ischemia/reperfusion. Hepatology. 2004;**39**:688-698. DOI: 10.1002/hep.20089

[41] Casillas-Ramírez A, Ben Mosbah I, Ramalho F, Rosello-Catafau J, Peralta C. Past and future approaches to ischemia-reperfusion lesion associated with liver transplantation. Life Sciences. 2006;**79**:1881-1894. DOI: 10.1016/j.lfs.2006.06.024

[42] Ben Mosbah I, Alfany-Fernández I, Martel C, Zaouali M, Bintanel-Morcillo M, Rimola A, et al. Endoplasmic reticulum stress inhibition protects steatotic and non-steatotic livers in partial hepatectomy under ischemia-reperfusion. Cell Death & Disease. 2010;**1**:e52. DOI: 10.1038/cddis.2010.29

[43] Bahde R, Spiegel H. Hepatic ischaemia-reperfusion injury from bench to bedside. The British Journal

of Surgery. 2010;**97**:1461-1475. DOI: 10.1002/bjs.7176

[44] Zúñiga J, Cancino M, Medina F, Varela P, Vargas R, Tapia G, et al. N-3 PUFA supplementation triggers PPAR-α activation and PPAR-α/NF-κB interaction: Anti-inflammatory implications in liver ischemia-reperfusion injury. PLoS One. 2011;**6**:e28502. DOI: 10.1371/journal.pone.0028502

[45] Ghonem N, Yoshida J, Stolz D, Humar A, Starzl T, Murase N, Venkataramanan R. Treprostinil, a prostacyclin analog, ameliorates ischemia-reperfusion injury in rat orthotopic liver transplantation. American Journal of Transplantation. 2011;**11**:2508-2516. DOI: 10.1111/j.1600-6143.2011.03568.x

[46] Kamo N, Shen X, Ke B, Busuttil R, Kupiec-Weglinski J. Sotrastaurin, a protein kinase C inhibitor, ameliorates ischemia and reperfusion injury in rat orthotopic liver transplantation. American Journal of Transplantation. 2011;**11**:2499-2507. DOI: 10.1111/j.1600-6143.2011.03700.x

[47] Broelsch C, Emond J, Whitington P, Thistlethwaite J, Baker A, Lichtor J. Application of reduced-size liver transplants as split grafts, auxiliary orthotopic grafts, and living related segmental transplants. Annals of Surgery. 1990;**212**:368-375

[48] Lo C, Fan S, Liu C, Lo R, Lau G, Wei W, et al. Extending the limit on the size of adult recipient in living donor liver transplantation using extended right lobe graft. Transplantation. 1997;**63**:1524-1528

[49] Arias-Diaz J, Ildefonso JA, Muñoz JJ, Zapata A, Jiménez E. Both tacrolimus and sirolimus decrease Th1/Th2 ratio, and increase regulatory T lymphocytes in the liver after ischemia/reperfusion. Laboratory Investigation. 2009;**89**:433-445. DOI: 10.1038/labinvest.2009.3

[50] Toso C, Patel S, Asthana S, Kawahara T, Girgis S, Kneteman NN, Shapiro AM, Bigam DL. The impact of sirolimus on hepatocyte proliferation after living donor liver transplantation. Clinical Transplantation. 2010;**24**:695-700. DOI: 10.1111/j.1399-0012.2009.01159.x

[51] Shinke H, Hashi S, Kinoshita R, Taniguchi R, Sugimoto M, Matsubara K, Ogawa E, Sonoda M, Takada N, Yoshizawa A, Ogawa K, Okamoto S, Uemoto S, Masuda S. Effectiveness of sirolimus in combination with cyclosporine against chronic rejection in a pediatric liver transplant patient. Biological & Pharmaceutical Bulletin. 2013;**36**:1221-1225

[52] Guillaud O, Gurram KC, Puglia M, Lilly L, Adeyi O, Renner EL, Selzner N. Angiotensin blockade does not affect fibrosis progression in recurrent hepatitis C after liver transplantation. Transplantation Proceedings. 2013;**45**:2331-2336. DOI: 10.1016/j.transproceed.2013.01.067

[53] Marsman HA, Heger M, Kloek JJ, Nienhuis SL, ten Kate FJ, van Gulik TM. Omega-3 fatty acids reduce hepatic steatosis and consequently attenuate ischemia-reperfusion injury following partial hepatectomy in rats. Digestive and Liver Disease. 2011;**43**:984-990. DOI: 10.1016/j.dld.2011.07.009

[54] Ibrahim ES, Saleh SM, El Hoseeny M, El Shaarawy A. Effect of omega-3 on hepatic regeneration in adult living donors undergoing hepatic resections for liver transplantation: A randomized controlled trial. Journal of Critical Care. 2016;**31**:157-162. DOI: 10.1016/j.jcrc.2015.09.022.

Chapter 3

Use of Intraoperative Ultrasound (IOUS) in Liver Surgery

Ali I. Yahya

Abstract

Over the last many years, diagnostic imaging has grown from a state of infancy to a high level of maturity. The various imaging modalities were developed over the last 50 years. Ultrasonography is one of the valuable tools in diagnosis of many diseases for a long time. It replaced X-ray in the diagnosis of many different diseases. It is noninvasive and has no complications if used many times in the day even if it is safe during pregnancy. The use of ultrasonography was spread over the years in all branches of medicine. It is promptly used in emergency medicine. Its use was introduced during operations. It showed excellent results when used for the assessment of liver tumors either primary or secondary liver tumors during open surgery and laparoscopy. The use of high-frequency ultrasound probe intraoperatively will nullify the abdominal wall and bowel gas effects on the result.

Keywords: intra-opertive ultrasound, liver surgery

1. History of IOUS

In 1942, Neurologist Karl Dussik used ultrasound first time in the medical diagnosis of brain tumors.

In 1948, George D. Ludwig developed the A-mode ultrasound equipment to detect gallstones.

John J. Wild is known as the "father of medical ultrasound" for imaging tissue in 1949. Modern ultrasonic diagnostic medical scans are descendants of the equipment developed by him and his colleagues in the 1950s.

In 1957–1958, Ian Donald, professor of obstetrics and gynecology from Glasgow, invented the ultrasound machine and developed first time the use of ultrasound in obstetrics.

The use of ultrasound during operations which is called intraoperative ultrasound was started in 1960 [3]; however, it was not widely accepted in use because of limited experience and the quality of ultrasound machine. Bernard Sigel is the surgeon who first performed intraoperative ultrasound in biliary surgery; it was in 1979, and later in 1980, he started using IOUS in hepatobiliary surgery.

In 1980, intraoperative ultrasound became more popular and widely used in the field of hepatobiliary and pancreatic, vascular, and neurosurgery.

In 1990, the use of intraoperative ultrasound became widely used, especially in liver surgery. And in the mid-1990s, the use of intraoperative ultrasound became a routine use in hepatic surgery; introduction of probes for open and laparoscopic surgery also added much in addition to the utilization of color Doppler flow ultrasound. IOUS is used for the assessment of pancreatic lesions, blood vessel invasion, lymph node metastasis, and also biopsy. The use of intraoperative ultrasound adds a lot of information on the anatomy and pathology of the lesion to the surgeon when he is standing at the operation table and can change the decision of the surgical management.

2. Use of intraoperative ultrasound for liver diseases

Ultrasound is used for diagnosis and assessment of liver diseases mainly for tumors, like colonic metastasis since 1990 with the use of a transducer either linear or T-shaped 3.7 MHz.

Intraoperative ultrasound can be used during an open or laparoscopic surgery; each approach has a unique probe. The use of ultrasound where the probe is put directly on the liver with no skin and abdominal wall interferes with the picture of the liver tissue.

The use of IOUS in different diseases:

1. Benign liver diseases

2. Malignant liver tumors

2.1 Benign liver diseases

The liver is a very important intra-abdominal organ, which is involved in different diseases that either originate in the liver itself or by a lesion in another part of the body and involves the liver like hepatic metastasis of malignancy. There are benign liver diseases, which are diagnosed by imaging like ultrasound, computed tomography, and magnetic resonance imaging.

2.1.1 Use of IOUS added changes in treatment of different benign liver lesions

2.1.1.1 Hydatid liver disease

Intraoperative ultrasound is used in surgery for hydatid liver disease. It is used routinely in our hospital.

Once the abdomen is opened, we examined the liver manually for localization of the cysts, and defining the number, we use T-shaped ultrasound probe sterilized by glutaraldehyde and examine the liver with the team of our consultant surgeons who perform IOUS and had good training in ultrasound. We examine the number of the cysts and contents in relation to the blood vessels and bile ducts, and visible bile duct communication will be notified if it is visible. Intraoperative ultrasound is more superior and informative than CT and MRI for hepatic hydatid disease, and it is found of value in the following [6–12]:

1. Localization of the cyst in relation to major blood vessels and bile duct.

2. Helping in planning hepatotomy to reach deep-seated cysts.

3. Aspiration and injection of deep-seated cysts—pair technique.

4. Trans-choledochal hydatid cyst evacuation—this is a very rare operation that was done for a 20-year-old female patient admitted to Zliten Teaching Hospital with obstructive jaundice and with percutaneous ultrasound and MRI. The cause of obstructive jaundice was due to the daughter hydatid cyst coming

from the mother hydatid cyst which was a deep-seated hepatic hydatid cyst in segment VIII with communication to the bile duct which was cleared by MRCP (**Figures 1** and **2**). The surgery was performed to the patient with the use of IOUS. The common bile duct was opened, and the daughter cysts from the bile duct were removed with the help of IOUS the mother cyst was cleared from daughter cysts by approach through the communication with the bile duct, Endocyst was removed, and the residual cavity collapsed which is clearly seen by IOUS. A T-tube was put inside the common bile duct, and the patient was discharged and after 4 weeks she had a T-tube contrast study. The common bile duct was clear, there was no more cyst in the liver, and the patient was cured from the hepatic hydatid-induced obstructive jaundice (**Figure 3**).

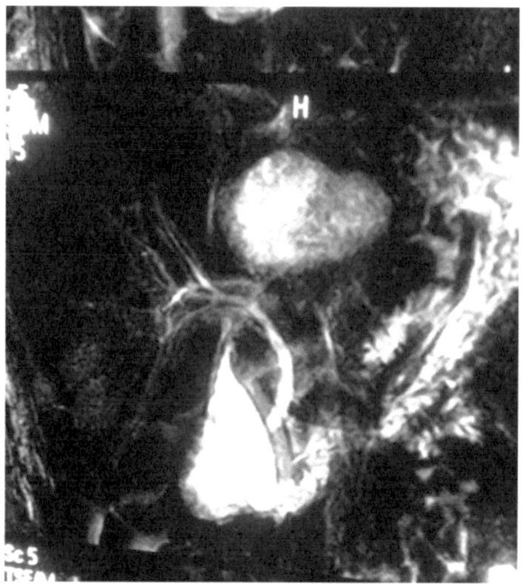

Hydatid cyst liver evacuated through bile duct.

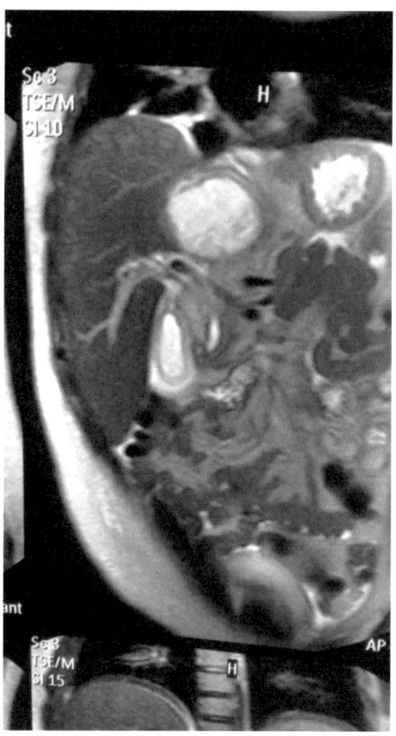

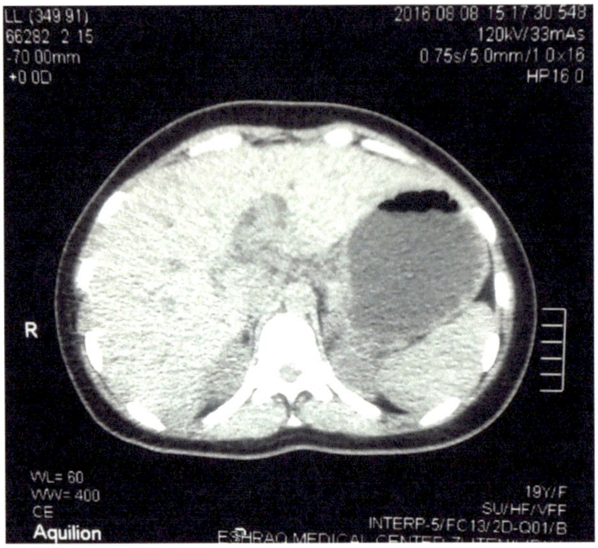

CT scan liver showing residual cyst was done after two months after the surgery

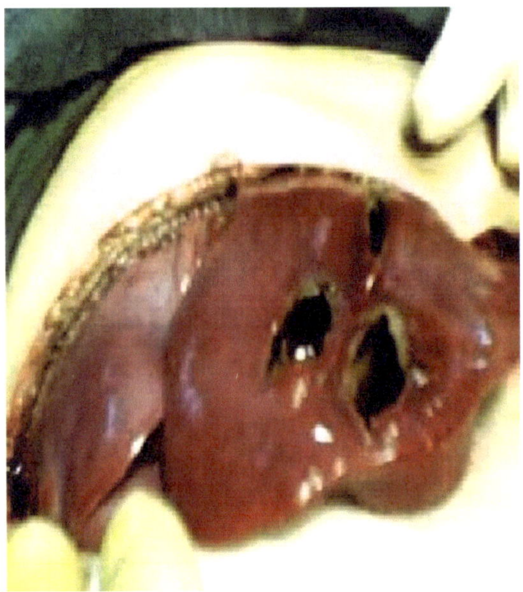

Figure 1.
Showing the liver with hydatid cysts in a child, aged 9 years, which had preoperative ultrasound which showed few hepatic hydatid cysts, with the use of intraoperative ultrasound; 22 hydatid cysts were removed in spite of the CT scan reporting few cysts.

2.1.1.2 Liver hemangioma

Liver hemangioma is not a common liver lesion; it can have a small size or may increase in size and rupture and can be detected by percutaneous ultrasound, CT, and MRI. Intraoperative ultrasound is used for delineation and plans the resection of the hemangioma. Hemangioma can be differentiated from other liver lesions by contrast-enhanced intraoperative ultrasound. It can be compressed under ultrasound and seen by Doppler, which is a feature of the space containing blood.

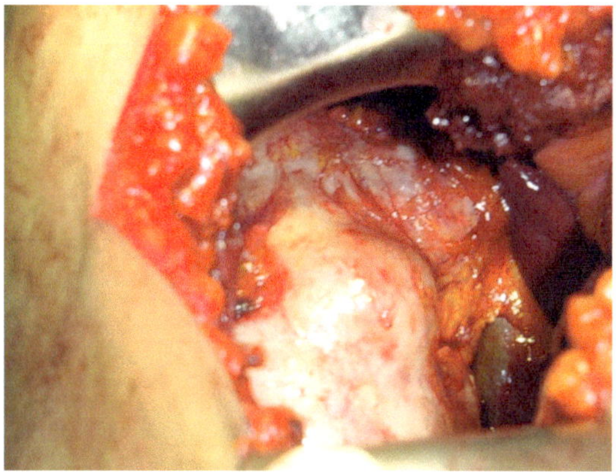

Figure 2.
Showing a patient with surgery for huge liver hydatid cyst. IOUS was used to scan the liver for other cysts and used in surgical approach to excise the cyst.

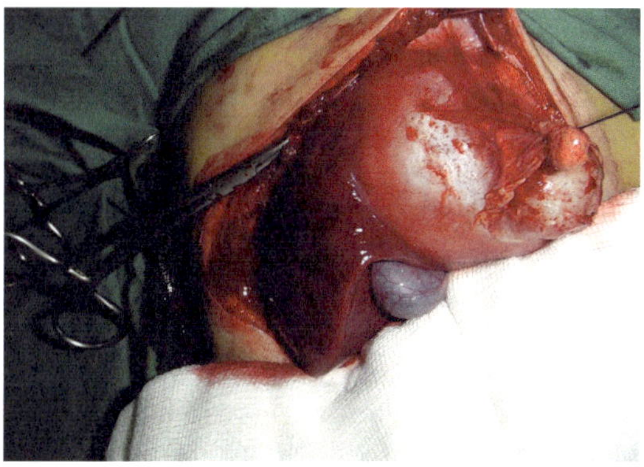

Figure 3.
Showing a big hydatid cyst in the liver.

2.1.1.3 Intraoperative ultrasound study of the gall bladder and the bile duct

With the development of transducers for intraoperative ultrasound, intrahepatic and extrahepatic bile ducts can be visualized with 7.5 MHz probes. We use T-shaped probes sterilized with glutaraldehyde solution or by gas sterilization; the probe can be covered with sterile sheet. Intraoperative laparoscopic ultrasound is used during laparoscopic cholecystectomy to visualize common bile lesions including stones, tumors, and gall bladder suspicious lesions either sludge or tumors.

Laparoscopic intraoperative ultrasound can replace intraoperative cholangiogram for the detection of common bile duct stones which costs less and consumes less time [1, 2, 4, 5] (**Figure 4**).

2.1.1.4 Liver cysts

Benign liver cyst, which can be congenital or acquired with the use of intraoperative ultrasound, we can delineate and study the relation of the cysts to the blood vessels and the bile duct.

2.1.1.5 Liver abscess

Liver abscess is not common; once happened it can be localized and aspirated with the help of intraoperative ultrasound.

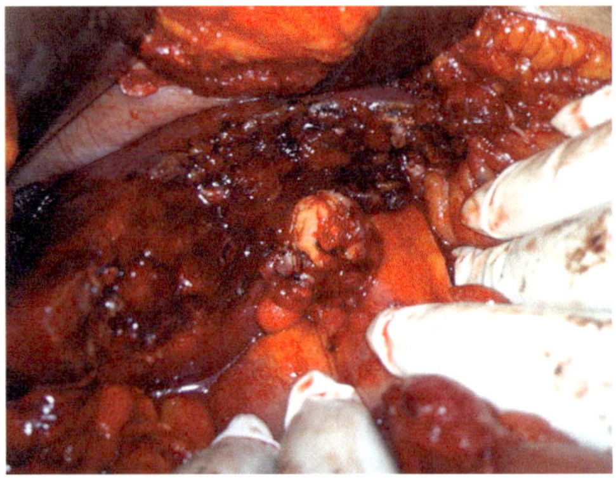

Figure 4.
A 60-year-old female patient with carcinoma in the gall bladder; the tumor was resected completely with segment of the liver.

2.1.1.6 Liver tumors

For primary liver tumors and hepatocellular carcinoma, IOUS is very helpful in staging the tumor looking for any small lesions. It is very helpful in case of a cirrhotic liver, l for looking the extent of the lesion, relation of the blood vessel to the lesion. It is more useful if contrast-enhanced ultrasound is used. IOUS is more superior in detecting liver lesion than preoperative MRI and CT scan with sensitivity of 95–100% in comparison to others, 80% for CT, and 70% for percutaneous ultrasound. It is very helpful in liver resection for liver malignant tumors and will improve patient survival by taking safety liver resection; with the use of IOUS, limited liver tumor resection can be done in a non-segmental way and will improve patient survival especially in a patient with hepatocellular carcinoma with a background of cirrhosis [25–27, 29–33]. IOUS may have difficulty in detecting small liver lesion in a fatty liver; however, the use of contrast-enhanced ultrasound will be more beneficial [22–24, 28].

For cholangiocarcinoma of the hilar region and Klatskin tumor, intraoperative ultrasound makes a difference in staging the disease and resection of the tumor.

Use of IOUS in malignant hepatic tumors:

1. IOUS scan for malignant liver lesions adds an outcome of 25–35% more over percutaneous ultrasound in liver resection and helps in defining the extent of the tumor and its relation to big blood vessels and the bile duct [13–21].

2. Helping in biopsy of liver lesions

The use of IOUS at primary surgery of colonic tumor is as follows: In our hospital it is done when the operation is performed by senior surgeons, and we found it gives more information on the staging of the tumor. It is found more superior than CT scan and percutaneous ultrasound.

2.1.1.7 Hepatic transplantation

It is used for harvesting the liver and for following the patency of anastomosis of the blood vessels.

3. IOUS

IOUS changed the surgical decision when used by hepatobiliary and pancreatic surgeons. The benefit of the use of IOUS in surgical treatment of a liver disease may reach to 41.9% according to documented studies and makes the use of IOUS for liver surgery of a big value.

3.1 IOUS training

1. Ultrasound is performed by the radiologist who had training and knowledge of operating on machines, and the radiologist and radiographer should be ready to perform the procedure in the right time.

2. It is difficult to perform IOUS during emergency operations, if needed.

3. Training of surgeons for the use of ultrasound during surgery needs time for different surgical operations.

3.2 Methods of the use of IOUS

1. Types of the transducer: the transducer can be for open surgery (linear or T-shaped). There are laparoscopic and robotic transducers which are used during laparoscopic surgery.

2. Sterilization: the transducer needs either sterilization or cover with sterile sheet to be used in surgery.

   Sterilization and disinfecting the probes:

   a. The transducer has to be cleaned after finishing the work and dried with dry tissue paper.

   b. Use the sterile sheet cover over the transducer, and put sterile gel during the examination inside the cover.

   c. Use a disinfective solution like CISEx; the time is 12 minutes. Glutaraldehyde and dialdehyde are not used nowadays because they may cause inflammatory contact.

   d. Hydrogen peroxide.

   e. Plasma.

3. Cover the ultrasound board with sterile sheet for the surgeon to use the board by himself.

4. Full mobilization of the liver by the removing of the ligaments before the application of IOUS.

5. Examining the remaining liver tissue for its blood flow and bile drainage. IOUS is a very crucial tool for modern liver surgery and changes the resection margin and the outcome.

6. When we examine the liver, we follow the portal veins and hepatic veins.

7. Looking for the pattern of the blood vessels: the flow of the blood, clotting in the blood vessels, and the pedicle supply of the resected and remaining segments.

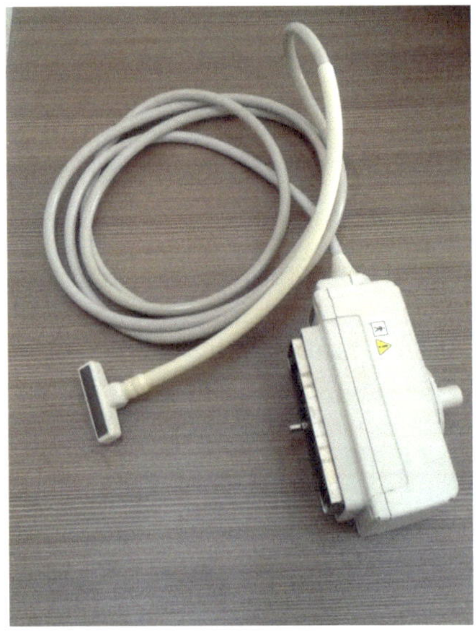

Open surgery ultrasound transducer

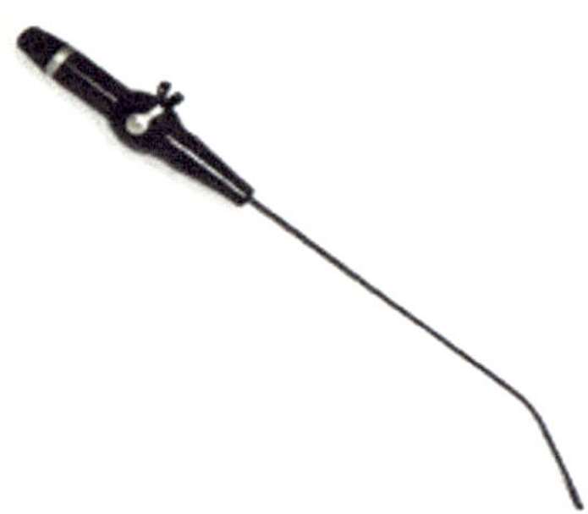

Laparoscopic ultrasound transducer

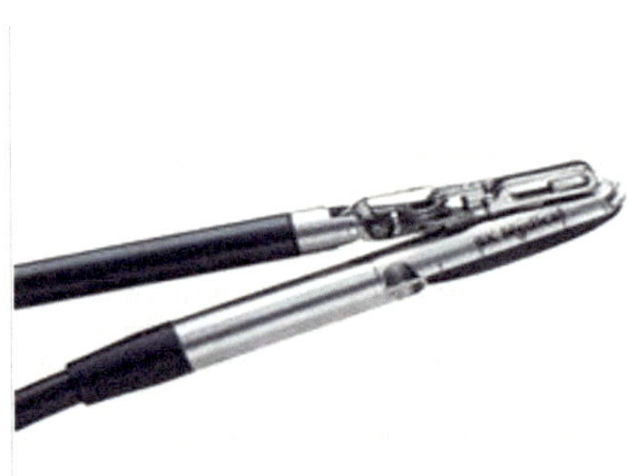

Robotic ultrasound transducer

4. Conclusion

Ultrasound is routinely used for the diagnosis of diseases. The use of ultrasound during surgery is applied for a long time, and it is used for surgical treatment of surgical liver diseases. It made a lot of changes in the management of malignant hepatic metastatic colonic tumors. Using IOUS for liver pathology will change the mode of treatment. It also helps in the ablation of liver tumors. IOUS is also used for surgical treatment of benign hepatic pathology like hydatid liver disease, liver cysts, bile duct stones, and bile duct tumors. It can replace intraoperative cholangiography when needed. The advantages of the use of IOUS in liver surgery are the following: it gives better informations about the liver involvement by the lesion than transcutaneous ultrasound, CT scan, or MRI; it will show small lesions which may not be seen by the other modalities; it helps in outlining the resection line when liver resection is planned; it gives informations about the relation of the blood vessels to the lesion; it gives information about the bile duct anatomy; and it can replace intraoperative cholangiogram if needed. Disadvantages of IOUS in liver surgery are the following: it needs special training for the surgeons, it adds more work for the radiologists if it needs to be done by the radiologist, and it is difficult to be used in emergency surgery like where patients are operated on malignant bowel obstruction to check whether the patient has liver metastasis or not. This is because of availability of the trained surgeon or trained radiologist and the availability of the equipment. The use of IOUS in liver surgery will add more cost, and it may not be possible in hospitals where the resources are restricted.

Author details

Ali I. Yahya
Zliten Teaching Hospital, Zliten Medical School, Al-Asmaria University, Zliten, Libya

*Address all correspondence to: aliyahyaz60@hotmail.com

References

[1] Lane RJ, Glazer G. Intra-operative B-mode ultrasound scanning of the extrahepatic biliary system and pancreas. Lancet. 1980;**2**:334-337

[2] Kolecki R, Schirmer B. Intra-operative and laparoscopic ultrasound. The Surgical Clinics of North America. 1998;**78**:251-271

[3] Kane RA. intraoperative ultrasonography: History, current state of the art, and future directions. Journal of Ultrasound in Medicine. 2004;**23**:1407-1420

[4] Sigel B, Machi J, Beitler JC, Donahue PE, Bombeck CT, Baker RJ, et al. Comparative accuracy of operative ultrasonography and cholangiography in detecting common duct calculi. Surgery. 1983;**94**(4):715

[5] Kruskal JB, Robert A. Intraoperative sonography of the biliary system. American Journal of Reotengraphy. 2001;**177**

[6] Botea F, Sârbu V, Dima S, Iusuf T, Unc O, Toldişan D, et al. The role of intraoperative ultrasound in the diagnosis and treatment of hydatid liver disease. Chirurgia (Bucur). 2006;**101**(6):593-598

[7] Ivanov SA, Kotiv BN. Ultrasound examination in the surgery of hepatic echinococcosis. Vestnik Khirurgii Imeni I. I. Grekova. 2001;**160**(3):73-77

[8] Gavrilin AV, Vishnevskiĭ VA, Ikramov RZ, Ambadi V. Intraoperative ultrasonic study in surgery of hepatic echinococcosis. Khirurgiia (Mosk). 1991;(2):78-82

[9] Picardi N, Annunziata A, Bartolacci M, Di Rienzo M, Bottegoni G, Zuccarini F, et al. The radical treatment of hepatic hydatidosis with deep and multiple locations. The role of new technologies particularly in the case of multiple locations. Annali Italiani di Chirurgia. 1999;**70**(4):529-538

[10] Dervisoglu A, Erzurumlu K, Taç K, Arslan A, Gürsel M, Hökelek M. Should intraoperative ultrasonography be used routinely in hepatic hydatidosis? Hepato-Gastroenterology. 2002;**49**(47):1326-1328

[11] Tasev V, Ionkov A. Intraoperative echography in the diagnosis and treatment of minor intraparenchymal cysts in multiple hepatic echinococcosis—A report on 3 cases. Khirurgia (Sofia). 1998;**51**(3):25-27

[12] Trotta F, Prati U, Roveda L, Brunetti E, Filice C. Intra-operative PAIR of hepatic echinococcal cyst after cholecystectomy with laparoscopic approach. Liver International. 2007;**27**(2):284-286

[13] Makuuchi M, Takayama T, Kosuge T, et al. The value of ultrasonography for hepatic surgery. Hepato-Gastroenterology. 1991;**36**:64

[14] Machi J, Isomoto H, Kurohiji T, et al. Accuracy of intraoperative ultrasonography in diagnosing liver metastasis from colorectal cancer: Evaluation with postoperative follow-up results. World Journal of Surgery. 1991;**15**:551

[15] Torzilli G, Olivari N, Moroni E, et al. Contrast-enhanced intraoperative ultrasonography in surgery for hepatocellular carcinoma in cirrhosis. Liver Transplantation. 2004;**10**(2 Suppl): S34-S38

[16] Castaing D, Emond J, Bismuth H, Kunstlinger F. Utility of operative ultrasound in the surgical management of liver tumors. Annals of Surgery. 1986;**204**:600-605

[17] Lau WY, Leung KL, Lee TW, Li AKC. Ultrasonography during liver resection for hepatocellular carcinoma. The British Journal of Surgery. 1993;**80**:493-494

[18] Garancini M, Gianotti L, Delitala A, Romano F, Degrate L, Giardini V. Intraoperative ultrasound: A review on its role in liver surgery for primitive and metastatic tumors. Minerva Chirurgica. 2016;**71**(3):201-213

[19] Donadon M, Costa G, Torzilli G. State of the art of intraoperative ultrasound in liver surgery: Current use for staging and resection guidance. Ultraschall in der Medizin. 2014;**35**(06):500

[20] Torzilli G, Makuuchi M. Tricks for ultrasound-guided resection of colorectal liver metastases. Hepato-Gastroenterology. 2003;**50**(49):1-3

[21] Meijer S, Paul MA, Cuesta MA, Blomjous J. Intra-operative ultrasound in detection of liver metastases. European Journal of Cancer. 1995;**31A**(7-8):1210-1211

[22] Mitsunori Y, Tanaka S, Nakamura N, Ban D, Irie T, Noguchi N, et al. Contrast-enhanced intraoperative ultrasound for hepatocellular carcinoma: High sensitivity of diagnosis and therapeutic impact. Journal of Hepato-Biliary-Pancreatic Sciences. 2013;**20**(2):234-242

[23] Arita J, Takahashi M, Hata S, Kokudo N. Usefulness of contrast enhanced intraoperative ultrasound using sonazoid in patients with hepatocellular carcinoma. Annals of Surgery. 2011;**254**(6):992-999

[24] Vazharov IP, Kostov DV. Intraoperative ultrasound examination OF hilar cholangiocarcinoma/tumor of klatskin. Journal of IMAB-Annual Proceeding (Scientific Papers). 2012;**18**. book 3

[25] Torzilli G, Del Fabbro D, Palmisano A, et al. Contrast-enhanced intraoperative ultrasonography during hepatectomies for colorectal cancer liver metastases. Journal of Gastrointestinal Surgery. 2005;**9**(8):1148-1153. discussion 1153-4

[26] Ferrero A, Langella S, Giuliante F, Viganò L, Vellone M, Zimmitti G, et al. Intraoperative liver ultrasound still affects surgical strategy for patients with colorectal metastases in the modern era. World Journal of Surgery. 2013;**37**(11):2655-2663

[27] van Vledder MG, Pawlik TM, Munireddy S, Hamper U, de Jong MC, Choti MA. Factors determining the sensitivity of intraoperative ultrasonography in detecting colorectal liver metastases in the modern era. Annals of Surgical Oncology. 2010;**17**(10):2756-2763

[28] Schulz A, Dormagen JB, Drolsum A, Bjørnbeth BA, Labori KJ, Kløw NE. Impact of contrast-enhanced intraoperative ultrasound on operation strategy in case of colorectal liver metastasis. Acta Radiologica. 2012;**53**(10):1081-1087

[29] Walker TLJ, Bamford R, Finch-Jones M. Intraoperative ultrasound for the colorectal surgeon: Current trends and barriers. Review article. ANZ Journal of Surgery. 2017;**87**(9):671-676

[30] Grondona P, Meola C, Floris F, Masini R, Brignole E, Quidaciolu F. Ultrasound-guided liver resection: Early experience in a district general hospital. Journal of Ultrasound. 2008;**11**(4):162-167

[31] Röthlin M, Schlumpf R, Bornman P, Krige J, Largiadèr F. Intraoperative

ultrasonography of the liver. Swiss Surgery. 1996;(3):105-111

[32] Torzilli G, Takayama T, Hui A-M, Kubota K, Harihara Y. A new technical aspect of ultrasound-guided liver surgery. The American Journal of Surgery. 1999;**178**(4):341-343

[33] Solomon MJ, Stephen MS, Gallinger S, White GH. Does intraoperative hepatic ultrasonography change surgical decision making during liver resection. The American Journal of Surgery. 1994;**168**(4):307-310

Chapter 4

Damage Control in Liver Surgery

Ali I. Yahya

Abstract

Damage control surgery is an old type of surgery practiced for many years to save the lives of badly injured patients. Damage control was first practiced in the American navy where a damaged vessel would receive minimal repair to keep it afloat. This translates to the field of medicine where minimal surgery is performed to save the life of a patient, and minimal action is taken to avoid major ailments, including hypothermia, acidosis, and coagulation defects during major trauma. Before World War II damage control surgery was popular, but later this type of surgery was abandoned. However, with a better understanding of the physiology of trauma and a revision of the outcome of badly injured patients, surgeons have reverted to damage control surgery, for example the packing of bleeding organs such as the liver and the controlling of sepsis, rather than taking patients to intensive care for further assessment. Damage control surgery has many benefits for badly injured patients and improves their chances of survival.

Keywords: liver trauma, perihepatic packing, acidosis, hypothermia, hypercoagulability

1. Definition of damage control

Damage control is defined as measures that are taken to minimize damage whether physical or non-physical. In emergency surgery it is the immediate action taken to stop bleeding and/or minimize sepsis, rather than taking the patient to intensive care for assessment. Damage control was first practiced in the American navy where a damaged vessel would receive minimal repair to keep it afloat.

2. History of damage control surgery

In ancient times, Greek and Roman physicians tried to use different modalities available at the time to save the lives of patients bleeding to death due to traumatic and non-traumatic causes. Millions of patients die around the world from bleeding each year. The liver packing technique, a highly effective technique to control bleeding, has been used in surgery for more than 100 years, where gauze packing is placed inside the liver wound to control the bleeding. Organ packing was used before World War II to control bleeding from liver wounds. Perihepatic packing goes back to 1908 when James Hogarth Pringle was the first surgeon to perform packing to stop massive bleeding from damaged liver at the Royal Glasgow Infirmary [1–3]. In 1913, Halstead used a rubber sheet between the gauze packs and the damaged liver tissue. After World War II, liver packing for a massively bleeding liver fell into decline. During the war the number of trauma patients with liver injury had intrahepatic packing to stop the bleeding. Trauma surgeons reported complications due to packing such as bleeding and abscesses, and since the war packing has been banned. From 1955 onwards, Madding, Lucas, and Ledgerwood performed liver packing on their patients and achieved good results. In 1981, David Felaciano performed liver packing on his patient [3], which gave potential results. In 1983, Harlan Stone was the first surgeon to follow damage control surgery by minimizing emergency surgery on exsanguinating patients from bleeding trauma due to a coagulation system defect [4], and performed periorgan packing, terminating the surgery on those unwell patients [5–7]. With the development of surgery and a better understanding of the physiology and pathology of trauma with different multicenter studies on the outcome of hepatic trauma, trauma surgeons reverted to the practice of ancient surgeons and used packing for bleeding organs. The decision to undertake damage control surgery should be decided as early as possible before the patient succumbs to the lethal triangle of acidosis, hypercoagulability, and hypothermia. By using damage control, 5 to 65% of patients may be controlled by packing. In 1970, no patients with uncontrolled massive liver injury were being treated with packing. In 1993, Rotondo and Schwab used the term damage control for the packing of bleeding organs [8–10]. Peitzman reported good results with damage control for major liver injury. Packing followed by angioembolization has produced excellent results [11]. Asensio had excellent experience with damage control surgery and produced excellent work in this regard. From 1990 to 2000, damage control was successfully applied in the management of severe abdominal trauma.

3. Stages of damage control surgery

Damage control surgery for patients with trauma or other non-traumatic surgery goes in danger of life if complete surgery. There are indications for damage control surgery, for example absolute indications and relative indications; however, it is better not to wait for indications.

Absolute indications include the following:

1. Acidosis, where the pH is less than 7.2.

2. Deranged clotting, where the patient bleeds, prolonged prothrombin time, and activated partial thromboplastin time.

3. Hypothermia, where the patient's temperature is less than 34°C.

These indications should be prevented [12].

Relative indications

1. Major intra-abdominal bleeding, which is very difficult to control.

2. Low blood pressure, where the carotid artery is weak or not palpable, systolic blood pressure is less than 70 mmHg, and tachycardia is evident.

3. Prolongation of time to control the bleeding is over 90 min.

4. Association with extra-abdominal injury.

5. Transfusion with more than 10 units of blood.

Stage I of damage control surgery is where the patient is taken to the operating theater and undergoes minimal and necessary surgical operations [13–15]. The above three usual causes following injury are leading causes of death in patients.

Massive transfusion, acidosis, and hypothermia have been considered as significant contributors to deranged clotting and coagulation manifestations. Hypothermia is caused by keeping the abdomen open for a long time, cold intravenous fluid, and blood. Acidosis happens due to low cardiac output. Tissue hypoxia techniques may include:

1. Removing a bleeding spleen or kidney.
2. Resection of devitalized bowel injury without performing anastomosis.
3. Packing a bleeding liver/packing a bleeding area.
4. Inserting vascular shunts.
5. Leaving the abdomen opened to prevent abdominal compartment syndrome

Stage II of damage control consists of:

- Admitting the patient to the intensive care unit, where the patient should be kept on a ventilator with complete relaxation and analgesia.
- Correcting for acidosis.
- Correcting for clotting by giving fresh frozen plasma and fresh blood.
- Correcting for hypothermia by warming both the patient and the fluid.
- Preventing complications such as infection, deep vein thrombosis, and adult respiratory distress syndrome (ARDS), which may happen in the intensive care unit.

Stage III of damage control ensures that once the patient is hemodynamically stable, he or she should be taken to the operating theater again within 24–72 h where the following procedures can be performed: removal of abdominal packs, removal of devitalized tissue, anastomosis of bowel, removal of shunts and performing vascular anastomosis, performing feeding jejunostomy, and closure of the abdominal wound.

4. Complications of damage control surgery

Intra-abdominal hypertension and abdominal compartment syndrome are the main and most serious complications of abdominal damage control surgery where intra-abdominal pressure rises above the normal level, which is 12 mmHg, and where the intra-abdominal pressure rises above 20 mmHg, which will affect the arterial perfusion pressure and result in organ dysfunction or failure; the condition will be labeled as abdominal compartmental syndrome. The following vital organs will be affected: kidneys, heart, lungs, liver, and gastrointestinal system. Its incidence ranges from 14% in patients with severe abdominal trauma to 50% in patients with severe trauma where the intra-abdominal pressure is above 12 mmHg. Perfusion of the vital organs is affected by intra-abdominal pressure (organ perfusion pressure = mean arterial pressure – intra-abdominal pressure). Once the intra-abdominal pressure is raised, perfusion to the vital organs will be decreased. The increase in intra-abdominal pressure is due to tissue edema; this edema could be bowel wall edema or edema of any intra-abdominal tissue, fluid overload by resuscitation, or capillary leakage because of inflammatory mediators released during trauma/sepsis.

5. Physiological effects of abdominal compartment syndrome

1. **Renal function**: because of the increase in intra-abdominal pressure, organ perfusion pressure will be reduced and renal blood flow will be reduced; glomerular filtration rate is reduced and urine output will decrease; the patient will suffer renal failure.

2. **Cardiac function**: increased intra-abdominal pressure will compress the vena cava and will result in reduced venous return; cardiac output will be reduced.

3. **Lungs function**: increased intra-abdominal pressure will result in reduced diaphragmatic movement, and will cause hypoventilation, increased airway pressure, and reduced lung compliance. All will end with hypoxia and hypercapnia, and because of sepsis and fluid overload will cause acute lung injury (ARDS). Prolonged lying down in the intensive care unit will be accompanied by deep vein thrombosis and can be followed by pulmonary embolism.

4. **Liver function**: hepatic blood flow will be reduced, impaired metabolism of glucose, lactate.

5. **Gastrointestinal function**: because of increased intra-abdominal pressure, bowel perfusion is reduced, and there will be bacterial translocation.

6. **Central nervous system function**: increased intra-abdominal pressure will cause a rise in intrathoracic pressure and increased central venous pressure will cause increased intracranial pressure and reduced cerebral perfusion pressure.

Forms of intra-abdominal pressure can be measured as follows:

1. Urinary bladder pressure, which is best measured by Foley's catheter.

2. Gastric pressure measured by nasogastric tube.

3. Trans-peritoneal needle connected to a monitor or manometer will detect intra-abdominal pressure.

4. Colonic pressure. Intra-abdominal hypertension is measured in grades:
   Grade I when the pressure is 12–15 mmHg.
   Grade II when the pressure is 16–20 mmHg.

Grade III when the pressure is from 21 to 25 mmHg.
Grade IV when the pressure is above 25 mmHg.
The incidence of abdominal compartment syndrome among severe trauma patients ranges from 1 to 14%.

Clinical presentation:

1. Pale-looking body color and hypotension.

2. Oliguria.

3. Breathlessness.

4. Abdominal distension.

5. Raised jugular venous pressure.

6. Peripheral edema.

Investigations:

No specific investigations, only clinical suspicion, measuring the abdominal pressure, and X-ray of the abdomen will show distension of bowel loops; a CT scan will show bowel wall edema.

Treatment of abdominal compartment syndrome:
It is better prevented than treated.

1. Urgent release of abdominal compartment tension by celiotomy.

2. Ventilator support.

3. Analgesia.

When applying damage control surgery in trauma patients, it is advisable to leave the abdomen open.

Management of open abdominal wound in cases of damage control surgery:

1. To avoid onset of compartment syndrome the abdominal wall should be left completely open or there should be partial approximation of the wound edges or skin only. If the abdomen is left completely open, the patient should be kept on a ventilator and completely paralyzed to avoid eviceration of the bowel outside the abdomen [16]. A plastic bag can be fixed to the edges of the abdomen wall with continuous stitches or skin clips like a sterile urine bag; towel clips, zipper sheath, and surgical mesh can also be used. This type of dressing allows the clinician to inspect the viscera, does not lead to increased intra-abdominal pressure, will not adhere to the bowel, and will be easier to remove. Once the patient improves and abdominal pressure is back to normal the abdominal wound can be closed. The patient may develop an incisional hernia, which can be dealt with later.

2. Intra-abdominal sepsis, because of the presence of gauzes inside the abdomen, will cause bacterial overgrowth. Major trauma may also be associated with bowel injury and contamination. Prolonged manipulation surgery and blood transfusion will also enhance bacterial overgrowth.

3. Missed organ injury like bowel injury if not recognized will result in a fistula between the bowel and the abdominal wall.

4. Bowel obstruction may be because of major surgery and gauzes left for some time. The bowel will stick at the inflammatory site and will result in bowel obstruction.

5. Hernia (abdominal wall hernia) may develop because of multiple surgeries and the abdomen being left open, resulting in weakness of the abdominal wall.

6. A longer stay in hospital or the intensive care unit may be inevitable.

7. Bile leak, collection of bile, and hemobilia may occur.

8. Vascular complications include hemorrhage, arteriovenous fistula, pseudoaneurysm and occur in 20–45% of patients with grade III to IV injury.

9. Bed sores can result from prolonged stays in the intensive care unit.

Figures 1–3 show a patient who had damage control laparotomy for intra-abdominal bleeding, where the abdomen was not closed.

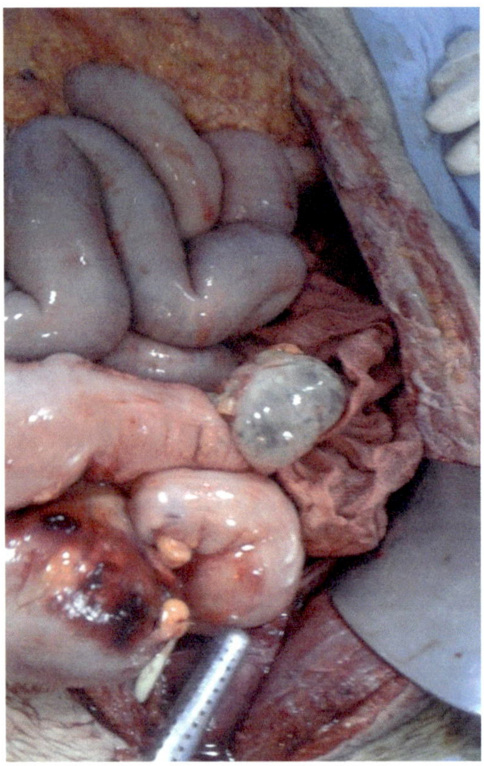

Figure 1.
Patient after major abdominal trauma, where the abdomen is left open.

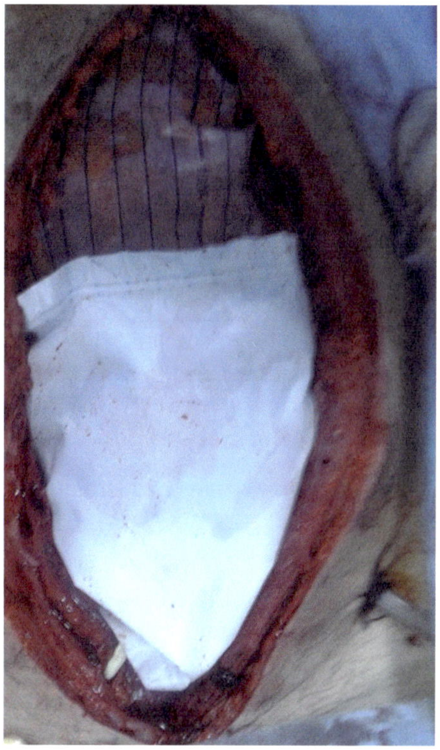

Figure 2.
Patient after major abdominal trauma, where the abdomen is closed with the use of a sterile plastic sheath, where we used sterile urine bag.

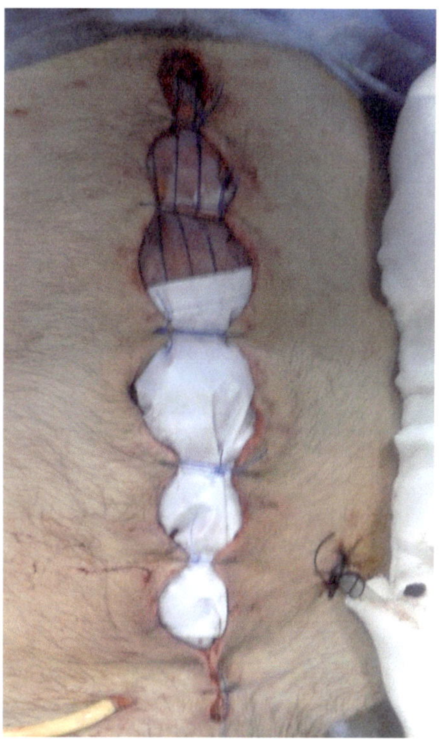

Figure 3.
The wound is approximated and not closed completely.

6. Benefits of damage control surgery

Damage control surgery is self-explanatory and it shows a big change in emergency surgery management. It has benefits for patient management:

1. Patients with massive uncontrolled hemorrhage can be saved from death by following the stages of damage control surgery, and the three biggest risks to patients are acidosis, hypothermia, and coagulopathy.

2. Mortality and morbidity can both be reduced.

3. A massively bleeding organ can be packed and the patient can be booked for another session of surgery where correction of acidosis, hypothermia, and coagulopathy can be performed, where the patient can be shifted to a tertiary center for surgery by a more qualified team [8].

4. Surgery can be deferred until an experienced surgeon is available, for example in places of combat.

7. Zliten Teaching Hospital's experience with damage control surgery

Zliten is a busy teaching hospital and provides medical and surgical treatment and nursing care for general and injured patients. It was heavily workloaded with injured people during the Libyan war in 2011 and is still receiving patients associated with weapon injury, in addition to other traumas such as road traffic accidents. In 1991, an 18 years-old Libyan, the first patient who had received perihepatic packing after severe liver injury grade IV, developed renal impairment, liver impairment, pleural effusion, and intestinal obstruction. He survived with major multiorgan insult and now is a medical doctor. The operative mortality of damage control is approximately 12% in Zliten hospital (**Figures 4–6**).

8. Experience of Zliten Teaching Hospital with damage control surgery

This experience was gained over a period of 27 years from 1991 to 2018. The number of patients with liver trauma is 324, with a female to male ratio of 26:298.

Most of the patients are between 20 and 40 years of age. Patient statistics are as follows:

Over 27 years, before the war, during the war, and after the war the number of patients with major liver trauma: 324.

Number of patients with perihepatic packing: 96.

Patients who survived after packing: 88.

Patients who died during packing and after packing: 8.

Patients who had the packs removed after 72 h: 76.

Patients who had repacking after 24 h: 4.

Patients who had packing removed at 48 h: 8.

Packing for non-trauma intra-abdominal bleeding: 5 patients.

Packing bleeding after hydatid liver surgery: 1 patient.

Massive bleeding postcholecystectomy with retrohepatic varices: 1 patient.

Massive bleeding after hepatic artery injury during postcholecystectomy: 1 patient.

Intragastric packing for gastropathy: 1 patient.

Intraurinary bladder packing for bleeding from prostatic tumor: 1 patient.

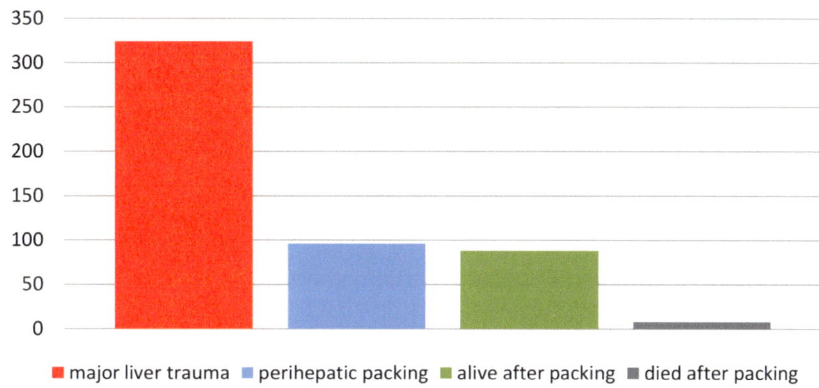

Figure 4.
Diagram showing major liver trauma at Zliten Teaching Hospital over a period of 27 years.

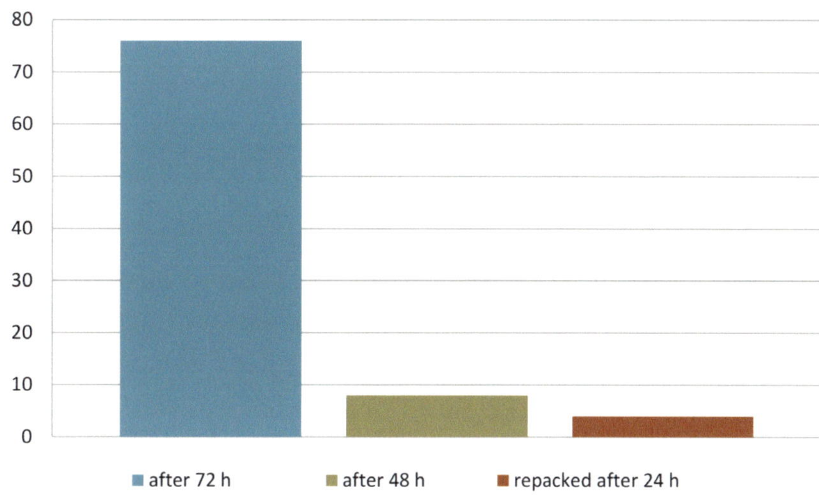

Figure 5.
Removal of the packs.

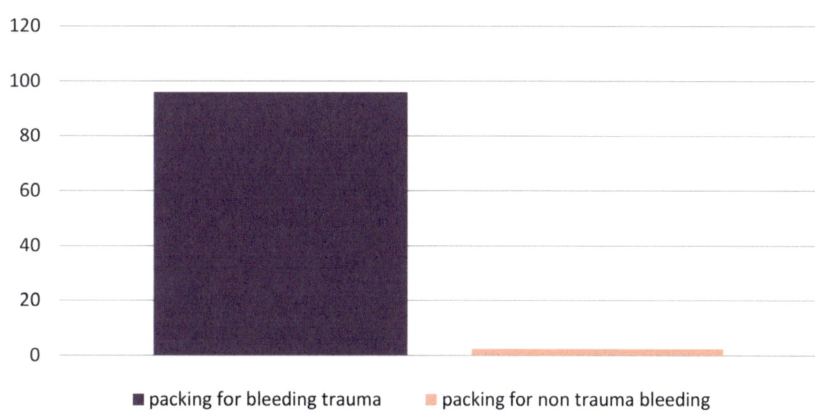

Figure 6.
Packing for trauma and non trauma intra-abdominal bleeding.

Complications after damage control surgery noticed among patients:

1. Bile leak: 4 patients stopped by themselves.
2. Wound dehiscence: 3 patients.
3. Bowel obstruction: 2 patients.
4. Postoperative jaundice: 3 patients due to massive transfusion.
5. Renal impairment: 1 patient.
6. Intra-abdominal abscess: 1 patient.
7. Intra-abdominal compartment syndrome: 4 patients.

Author details

Ali I. Yahya
Zliten Teaching Hospital, Zliten Medical School, Al Asmaria University, Zliten, Libya

*Address all correspondence to: aliyahyaz60@hotmail.com

References

[1] Leppaniemi A. Who invented damage control surgery? Scandinavian Journal of Surgery. 2014;**103**:165-166

[2] Lin B-C, Fang J-F, Ray-Jade Chen R-J, Yon-Cheong Wong Y-C, Yu-Pao Hsu Y-P. Laparotomy with perihepatic packing in one trauma centre. Injury. 2014;**45**(1):122-127

[3] Roberts DJ, Ball CG, Feliciano DV, Moore EE, Ivatury RR, Lucas CE, et al. History of the innovation of damage control for management of trauma patients: 1902-2016. Annals of Surgery. 2017;**265**(5):1034-1044. DOI: 10.1097/SLA.0000000000001803

[4] Holcomb JB, Jenkins D, Rhee P, Johannigman J, Mahoney P, Mehta S, et al. Damage control resuscitation: Directly addressing the early coagulopathy of trauma. The Journal of Trauma: Injury Infection and Critical Care. 2007;**62**(2):307-310

[5] Benz D, Balogh ZJ. Damage control surgery: Current state and future directions. 2017;**23**(6):491-497

[6] Weber DG, Bendinelli C, Balogh ZJ. Damage control surgery for abdominal emergencies. The British Journal of Surgery. 2014;**101**(1):e109-e118

[7] Paydar S, Mahmoodi M, Jamshidi M, Niakan H, Keshavarz M, Moeenvaziri N, et al. Perihepatic packing versus primary surgical repair in patients with blunt liver trauma; an 8-year experience. Bulletin of Emergency and Trauma. 2014;**2**(3):103-109

[8] Doklestić K, Djukić V, Ivančević N, Gregorić P, Lončar Z, Stefanović B, Jovanović D, Karamarković A. Severe blunt hepatic trauma in polytrauma patient—Management and outcome. Srpski Arhiv za Celokupno Lekarstvo. 2015;**143**(7-8):416-422

[9] Cirocchi R, Abraha I, Montedori A, Farinella E, Bonacini I, Tagliabue L, et al. Damage control surgery for abdominal trauma. Cochrane Database of Systematic Reviews. 2010;**20**(1):CD007438. DOI: 10.1002/14651858.CD007438.pub2

[10] Germanos S, Gourgiotis S, Villias Marco Bertucci C, Dimopoulos N, Salemis N. Damage control surgery in the abdomen: An approach for the management of severely injured patients. International Journal of Surgery. 2008;**6**(3):246-252

[11] Dabbs DN, Stein DM, Scalea TM. Major hepatic necrosis: A common complication after angioembolization for treatment of high-grade liver injuries. The Journal of Trauma. 2009;**66**(3):621-627

[12] Rotondo MF, Schwab CW, McGonigal MD, Phillips GR 3rd, Fruchterman TM, Kauder DR, et al. "Damage control": An approach for improved survival in exsanguinating penetrating abdominal injury. The Journal of Trauma. 1993;**35**(3):375-382

[13] Di Saverio S. Predictive factors of morbidity and mortality in grade IV and V liver trauma undergoing perihepatic packing: Single institution 14 years experience at European Trauma Centre. Injury—International Journal of the Care of the Injured. 2012;**43**(9):1347-1354

[14] Beuran M, Iordache FM. Damage control surgery—New concept or reenacting of a classical idea? Journal of Medicine and Life. 2008;**1**(3):247-253

[15] Sharrock AE, Midwinter M. Damage control—Trauma care in the first

hour and beyond: A clinical review of relevant developments in the field of trauma care. Annals of the Royal College of Surgeons of England. 2013;**95**(3):177-183

[16] Ng N, McLean SF, Ghaleb MR, Tyroch AH. Hepatic "BOLSA" a novel method of perihepatic wrapping for hepatic hemorrhage, "BOLSA". International Journal of Surgery Case Reports. 2015;**13**:99

Section 3

Types of Hepatic Surgery

Chapter 5

Standard Open Right Hepatectomy

Luis Cesar Bredt

Abstract

The evolution of hepatic resection from an imprecise removal of portions of the liver often associated with a mortality rate of up to 20% to a routine and controlled anatomic procedure with operative risk less than 5%, represents a major advance in modern surgery. This accomplishment has been made thanks to better understanding of the liver vascular and biliary anatomy, recognition of the functional reserve of the liver and the potential for regeneration, advances is surgical technique as well as anesthesia and perioperative care. These factors, along with the improvement of prolonged survival following hepatic resection for colorectal metastases, hepatocellular and cholangiocarcinoma have led to an expansion of liver surgery. In this chapter, we will give the evolution of the technique used for the standard open right hepatectomy. In addition, we will describe on detail our technique employed for right hepatectomy focusing on indications, preoperative preparation and specific technical aspects.

Keywords: hepatectomy, open right, liver resection

1. Introduction

The evolution of hepatic resection from an imprecise removal of portions of the liver often associated with a mortality rate of up to 20% to a routine and controlled anatomic procedure with operative risk less than 5%, represents a major advance in modern surgery. This accomplishment has been made thanks to better understanding of the liver vascular and biliary anatomy, recognition of the functional reserve of the liver and the potential for regeneration, advances is surgical technique as well as anesthesia and perioperative care. These factors, along with the improvement of prolonged survival following hepatic resection for colorectal metastases, hepatocellular and cholangiocarcinoma have led to an expansion of liver surgery.

In this chapter, we will give the evolution of the technique used for the standard open right hepatectomy. In addition, we will describe on detail our technique employed for right hepatectomy focusing on:

- Indications
- Preoperative preparation
- Specific technical aspects

2. Surgical anatomy

It was the work from our center conducted by Bismuth [1] which introduced to the English speaking word, the segmental approach to liver surgery, which in turn was based on the anatomical description of the liver by Couinaud [2]. The two liver lobes are divided into four segments with defined blood inflow and outflow as well as biliary drainage. The fibrous Glissonian sheath surrounds the branches of the segmental structures, whereas the hepatic veins lie between the pairs of the liver segments [3, 4].

For further details on liver anatomy of interest for surgeons performing liver surgery the reader is referred to the chapter on liver anatomy on this book.

3. Indications

Currently, hepatic and right liver resections may be required in a wide variety of conditions, including pathological processes which are limited to the respective right side of the liver. Partial right hepatectomy in the treatment of primary (benign or malignant) liver tumors, biliary tract tumors and secondary malignant tumors are the most common indications. Partial right hepatic resections may also be necessary in the management of complex cystic diseases, benign biliary stenoses, some hepatic trauma, and more recently in liver transplantation with live donors. Total hepatectomies are reserved for situations of liver uptake in cadaveric donors and hepatic replacement in the hepatic transplant recipient.

4. Different techniques of hepatectomy

The modern era of anatomic resection dates as far back as 1950s, when Lortat-Jacob [5] reported the technique of right hepatectomy by performing an initial dissection, ligation and division of the right hepatic artery, portal vein and right hepatic vein, followed by parenchyma transection with intrahepatic isolation of the vessels. Although, this technique is advantageous as it reduces the bleeding during the parenchyma transection in addition to displaying the demarcation line between healthy and ischemic parenchyma, it is associated with serious complications such as major bleeding and air embolism (if the right hepatic vein is injured during the dissection of its non-parenchymal route). For this reason, Lortat-Jacobs' original technique [5], was later modified by preceding the portal and hepatic vein dissection by supra- and infra-hepatic caval control. This technique has, however, two drawbacks: firstly, the already mentioned risk of trauma to the hepatic vein, and secondly, the possibility of devascularization of parts of remaining liver in cases of anatomical variations. In addition, during a right hepatectomy, the extrahepatic ligation of the right pedicle is associated with a risk of ligation of the biliary convergence situated anterior to the origin of the right portal branch.

In contrast, these complications are less frequent with the technique described by Tung and Quang [6] which entails an initial parenchymal dissection with intrahepatic control of the vessels.

Although, other techniques have been described, generally most liver surgeons use a combination of these techniques often applied in accordance to case specifics.

The technique we use, first described by Bismuth [7], consists of an initial hilar dissection to control the arterial and portal components without touching the biliary duct (**Figure 1**).

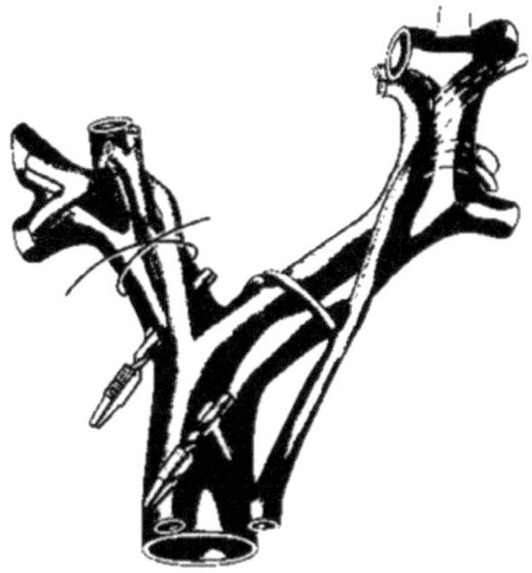

Figure 1.
Control of the arterial and portal components without touching the biliary duct.

The control of right hepatic vein can also be done at this stage, however, this is not essential and should be avoided if difficulties are anticipated. This technique has the advantage of preceding the parenchymal section by the selective control of the right arterioportal and right hepatic components (as in the technique described by Lortat-Jacob) [5] and tie the vessels in the hepatic parenchyma (as in the technique described by Ton That Tung) [6].

5. Preoperative evaluation

Before any decision to perform a major surgical procedure could be made there is a need for a thorough pre-operative evaluation of the patients focused on the general physical status as related to the requirements of the planed operative procedure. All factors needed for a proper evaluation of the risk and possible gain from the patient's point of view should be taken into account. In this aspect liver resection does not differ from any other major surgical resection. However, there are factors that are specific to liver resection: the risk for massive intraoperative hemorrhage and postoperative functional hepatic insufficiency. The preoperative evaluation of the functional capacity of the remaining liver is difficult and there are no strict and objective rules and specific knowledge and experience is required. In general, to determine the indications for surgery and the possible course of the prognosis following the surgical treatment, evaluation of liver cell integrity, excretory, and metabolic performance as well as the expected temporary ischemia and the effects of the anesthesia are all of importance [8]. Risk factors should be taken into account particularly fibrosis/cirrhosis or small future remnant volume and the question whether resection safety can be increased by portal vein embolization (PVE) should be examined preoperatively [9].

Also, the preoperative evaluation should aim at clarifying the following questions:

- The extent of the pathological lesions.
- Detailed evaluation of the pathological lesions within the hepatic parenchyma and the relationship with important structures such as vascular and biliary components.

In this regard, a three phase spiral computerized tomography (CT) and a magnetic resonance (MR) can be of a significant help. However, further information and accuracy with great clinical benefit during the preoperative evaluation is obtained from 3D CT or MR reconstruction, vascular reconstruction as well liver volume measurements.

6. Operative procedure

6.1 Installation

The patient is placed on supine position. The right arm is placed along the body wrapped in a drape whose ends pass under the back of the patient. The left arm is stretched at 90°. For anesthesiological monitoring, central venous lines and an arterial pressure sensor are placed. A gastric tube may be used to decompress the stomach.

The surgical field usually extends from the lower half of the chest to the pubic symphysis. The patient's head is turned to the right and fixed on this position by Elastoplast® tape in order to expose the left jugular triangle. The site of the abdominal incision is marked and the entire operative field is then covered. For large tumors requiring a thoracoabdominal incision or median sternotomy, the entire chest is included in the surgical field.

6.2 Surgical incision

An optimal surgical approach is a prerequisite for safe, controlled liver resection. For right hepatic resection, we use almost exclusively an abdominal approach. This involves a median incision with right transverse extension (**Figure 2**).

Depending on the case, the incision usually can be extended cranial over the xiphoid process. A bicostal incision may provide a very good exposure suitable for almost all types of standard hepatectomies.

Extension of the incision into the chest is exceptional, however, in extreme cases the incision can be extended further by a partial sternotomy, giving an excellent exposure of the suprahepatic vena cava. Similarly, a thoraco-phreno-laparotomy is used rarely for very large tumors of the right lobe or the upper right lobe preventing the mobilization and control of the suprahepatic vena cava.

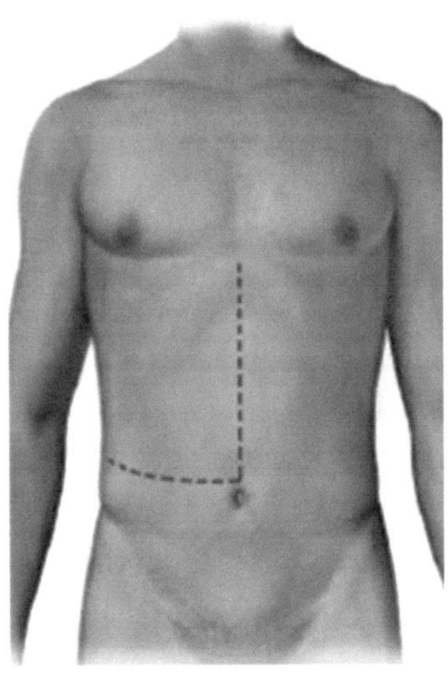

Figure 2.
Median incision with right transverse extension (modified Makuuchi incision).

6.3 Abdominal exploration

This step involves a complete exploration of the abdominal cavity paying special attention to the liver in order to identify possible undiagnosed lesions which could constitute a contraindication to liver resection. In general, it is possible to perform this step via a limited right subcostal incision. The first part of the exploration involves a manual palpation which is focused on the left liver, porta hepatis (in particular the lower posterior aspect) and the coeliac region. Division of the ligamentum teres and the falciform ligament along the anterior surface of the liver facilitates the exploration. The elevation of the ligamentum teres helps to expose the inferior surface of the liver and the area of the hilus as well as umbilical fissure. Performing this step (elevation of the ligamentum teres) helps to identify and better estimate lesions which can be potentially missed or underevaluated. Exploration should also include the inferior quadrants of the abdomen looking for adenopathy, peritoneal carcinomatosis or any lesion indicating colonic recurrence. Frozen section biopsies should be done for suspected lesions.

The second part of the exploration involves performing an ultrasound (US) examination of the liver. The US helps to identify previously undetected lesions and to clearly delineate anatomical landmarks in the relation to the tumor [10]. The intraoperative US is particularly beneficial for deep seated lesions <10 mm in diameter as identification of these lesions may influence the surgeon to change the strategy and/or tip the balance against a curative resection. In addition, US may identify anatomical variations that may make the resection more difficult, such as accessory hepatic veins or common origins of the portal pedicles [11]. Finally, ultrasound is an indispensable aid when the anatomy is altered by a previous hepatectomy. If the exploration (manual and by US) is negative, the incision is enlarged to start the mobilization of the liver.

6.4 Liver mobilization

Following the division of the ligamentum teres, the posterosuperior remaining part of the falciform ligament is incised and divided as far back as the suprahepatic IVC. The space between the right hepatic vein (RHV) and middle hepatic vein (MHV) is dissected 2 or 3 cm in the caudal direction. In a similar fashion, the perihepatic attachments (right and when required left coronary ligament) are divided. This begins from the right lateral side and continues to the inferior peritoneal reflection exposed by retracting the right lobe anterosuperiorly. During this stage it is important to stay in close contact to the liver surface so to avoid entering the retroperitoneum. Failure to do so may result on profuse bleeding from severed retroperitoneal veins, which at times can be very dilated, particularly in patients with portal hypertension. Similarly, after dividing the upper lamina of the coronary ligament, care should be taken not to enter the thickness of the diaphragm as it can cause bleeding which often requires a time consuming hemostasis. In addition, adhesions between liver and diaphragm when present should not be digitally dissected (especially with a cirrhotic liver) as this approach is associated with a real risk of liver decapsulation leading to massive bleeding.

Multiple short Spigelian veins between the IVC and posterior surface of the liver are ligated and divided as the liver is retracted anteriorly and laterally to the left. If an inferior right hepatic vein/s are present (>5 mm) it is crucial to ligate and divide them as they are a potential source of major bleeding. During this stage, one often encounters a band of ligamentous tissue extending from the liver to the right lateral aspect of the vena cava and in some patients this represents a small bridge of liver parenchyma. Regardless the nature, this too requires ligation and division as most of the time this band contains one or two veins.

After the right liver is fully mobilized, the space between the RHV and the MHV in the anteromedian surface of the vena cava is carefully dissected using a right angle forceps through which a tape is passed around to control the root of the RHV. Having achieved this, laparotomy pads are placed behind the liver to enhance the exposure of the right lobe necessary for the parenchyma resection.

It is not unusual that during mobilization to find right lobe tumors attached to the diaphragm. The surgeon should either separate these attachments or in some cases resect a segment of the diaphragm which can be subsequently repaired. Tumor attachment/s to the diaphragm should not be considered as distal metastatic lesions and should not influence the surgeon to abandon the planed resection.

6.5 Hilar dissection

After cholecystectomy, the right lateral aspect of the hepatoduodenal ligament is incised longitudinally just posterior to the bile duct, followed by a hilar dissection to identify and achieve control of the right hepatic artery (RHA) and right portal vein (RPV). The right hepatic artery is identified during the cholecystectomy. Anomalies such as having a right hepatic artery originating from the superior mesenteric artery or posterior location in the hepatoduodenal ligament should always be kept in mind if injuries are to be prevented. Ideally, these possibilities should be excluded during the preoperative work-up by CT angiography imaging. The artery is traced to its left sufficiently to identify with certainty its junction with the proper hepatic artery after which the right branch is controlled.

The next step involves the exposure of the portal vein. Using gently a blunt right angle forceps, the trunk of portal vein is dissected anteriorly and posteriorly and a traction tape is passed around this vessel. Dissection is then continued into the hilum of the liver to expose the bifurcation of the portal vein, where the right branch is freed up and controlled by a vascular tape. During this step, one should be careful to avoid two possible complications. First, the left portal vein tends to pass directly away from the operator and care must be taken not to injure it. Second, the possibility of small tributaries from the right portal branch to the caudate lobe should always be kept in mind as failure to do so may lead to cumbersome bleeding from such very fine veins. Hilar dissection is completed by tracing the common bile duct into the hilum where the right and left branches are seen. Insertion of a small catheter through the cystic duct stump and up into the left and right ducts can be useful to identify these structures as a preparation step for eventual division (during the parenchyma transection).

An initial occlusion of RHA and RPV with bulldog clamps will reveal a demarcation line on the liver surface that corresponds to the transection plane, which is marked with electrocautery. The isolation and clampage of the right arterial and portal branches is advantageous as it allows selective clamping without inducing ischemia in the contralateral site of the liver [12–14].

One important point to remember is that at the end of this step the surgeon has two options. First, as described above to dissect and control the vascular components (right hepatic and portal branch) followed by parenchyma transection. Second, to dissect, ligate and divide the vascular components before commencing the parenchymal transection. The choice will depend on the case particulars and on the surgeons' preference.

6.6 Parenchymal transection

After selectively controlling the right lobe inflow and outflow, transection of the parenchyma is commenced along the marked line running from an anteroinferior to posterosuperior direction near the diaphragmatic hiatus of the IVC for early exposure of the middle hepatic vein. The transection is done using either a Kelly clamp or ultrasonic dissector with selective occlusion of the vascular inflow (RHA and RPV). While the ultrasonic dissector is highly effective for exposure of the periportal pedicles, care must be taken with this instrument when dissecting in close contact to the hepatic veins whose walls are extremely fragile. In addition, one should be always aware of the location of the tumor to achieve a negative histologic margin. When the resection is performed in a fibrous or cirrhotic liver, using a small Kelly clamp (kellyclasie) to carry out the transection may be preferable. As parenchymal division proceeds, pedicles including the larger branches originating from the hepatic veins are tied with silk 4.0. We do not use metal clips or absorbable material to achieve the hemostasis in transection surface of the remaining parenchyma. In our experience, the clips can easily be removed/dislodged during manipulations, by vigorous suction or when the liver becomes very congested or edematous leading to unnecessary bleeding and time delay to control it.

Care must be taken to preserve the middle hepatic vein by carefully ligating its branches to the anterosuperior and anteroinferior segments of the right lobe and by preserving the venous drainage of the medial segment of the left lobe. The parenchyma is divided in an anteroposterior direction until the anterior surface of the IVC is exposed. Before the specimen is removed it is necessary to divide the right portal pedicle and right hepatic vein. The right hepatic artery already controlled is double ligated with nonabsorbable suture (Cardionyl® 4.0), whereas the portal vein is sutured transversely with Cardionyl® 5.0 in order to prevent stricture of the remnant portal trunk. At this stage, the right biliary duct as the only remaining anatomical structure of the pedicle is in turn divided and closed with PDS 6.0. The right hepatic vein as the last structure holding the specimen, clearly exposed by a combined approach (extrahepatic dissection above the liver and laterally along the vena cava as well as medially by the parenchymal transection) is double clamped using DeBakey clamps and divided leaving sufficient length to perform a secure closure with Prolene® 4.0, or it may be divided using a vascular stapler. Alternatively, the right hepatic vein can be controlled and divided intrahepatically during the parenchyma transection. However, extrahepatic control reduces blood loss as the liver is divided and is very important maneuver for tumors close to the vena cava. Following the removal of the specimen, it is important to check for possible bile leaks by injecting methylene blue either via the cystic duct stump or the stump of the right bile duct before closing it. Bile leaks on the resection surface are easily visualized and selectively closed by using monofilament sutures. With the described technique for the parenchymal transection, the cut surface is usually dry, however, when required the hemostasis is achieved by gentle manual compression combined sometimes with application of biological fibrin glues.

Following resection, torsion of the mobilized left lobe may occur which can potentially lead to either kinking of the vessels in the hilum or the left hepatic vein. By refixing the falciform ligament this complication can be prevented. In addition, the diaphragmatic veins, vena cava, the surface of the parenchyma, hepatic artery and the integrity of the bile duct are checked before abdominal closure.

6.7 Technical variations

6.7.1 The liver hanging maneuver

In 2001 Belghiti described a technique termed the "liver hanging manoeuvre" (LHM). In this procedure, the liver is lifted by a tape passed between the anterior surface of the vena cava and the liver, thereby providing effective vascular control, in order to make the anterior approach safer and easier [15].

The classic technique was first described to facilitate right hepatectomy by the anterior approach. In this first variant of the procedure, the anterior aspect of the suprahepatic IVC is exposed and the space between the right hepatic vein (RHV) and the middle hepatic vein (MHV) is dissected along the IVC axis for 2–3 cm, and when the dissection is complete, the hepatic parenchyma is looped up with a tape.

During the parenchymal transection, continuous upwards traction is applied on the tape by holding both its ends together. The tape ensures the safety of the underlying major vascular structures during transaction in a manner akin to dissecting on the finger to protect an important underlying structure. The tape elevates the liver, making it easier to transect, and constantly guides the surgeon towards the correct plane, thereby enabling a vertical transaction along the shortest possible route. The traction on the tape can also be regulated to provide control in instances of venous bleeding to help identify the vessel.

In "up to down" technique, the classic technique is modified in order to increase its security that no major bleeding occurs during the maneuver [16]. The entire blind dissection of the RHIVC tunnel is performed in a craniocaudal direction in order to avoid the possible risk of RHV or MHV injury by the clamp inserted caudally. The maneuver is begun between the RHV and MHV, this space usually does not contain SHVs [17], and can be safely dissected for 3–4 cm downwards with a right-angled vascular clamp without any risk. The long axis of the RHIVC does not always represent a straight perpendicular line, but may take a straight-oblique or slightly curved course [17]. For this reason the dissection should be performed along a right oblique axis rather than in vertical direction to reduce the risk of injury to the caudate processus vein.

6.8 Drainage

Drainage is carried out by silicone drains. Two drains are brought out on the lower edge of the surgical incision, one placed on the right subdiaphragmatic space near the resected surface, whereas the second drain whose end lies in the foramen of Winslow is placed under the liver. In general, we believe that hepatectomies should be drained as this measure reduces the risk of postoperative hematoma formation or bile collection.

7. Immediate operative care

The patient is kept in ICU for a minimum of 12 h in order to begin monitoring potential postoperative complications (**Table 1**).

• Bleeding • Post-hepatectomy liver failure • Biliary fistula • Post-operative ascites • Surgical infection • Coagulation disorders • Pulmonary infection and respiratory disorders • Acute kidney injury • Hepatorenal syndrome

Table 1.
Potential postoperative complications of right hepatectomy.

8. Final considerations

The adoption of a specific technique for right hepatectomy is related to the preference of the surgeon and for each specific situation, however, it is desirable that surgeons are familiar with various techniques available to perform the operation. An obvious example is the resection of large tumors of the right lobe in these cases and it is desirable, but impossible, to maintain the conventional mode of hepatic resection with mobilization of the wolf right prior to transection. Another example is the ability to promptly apply occlusion of vascular influx, or even total vascular exclusion, in case of bleeding during hepatectomy.

The surgical risks associated with hepatic resection are now smaller, especially in specialized centers and high volume liver operations.

Author details

Luis Cesar Bredt
Surgical Oncology and Hepatobiliary Surgery, University Hospital of Western Paraná, State University of Western Paraná, Cascavel, Paraná, Brazil

*Address all correspondence to: lcbredt@gmail.com

References

[1] Bismuth H. Les hépatectomies: Encycl méd.-Chir., Techniques Chirurgicales—Appareil Digestif. Paris: Editions Techniques Ed; 1968, 4.2.07, 40762

[2] Couinaud C. Le foie. Etudes Anatomiques et Chirurgicales. Paris: Masson Ed; 1957

[3] Goldsmith NA, Woodburne RI. Surgical anatomy pertaining to liver resection. Surgery, Gynecology & Obstetrics. 1957;**195**:310-318

[4] Launois B, Jamieson GG. The importance of Glisson's capsule and its sheaths in the intrahepatic approach to resection of the liver. Surgery, Gynecology & Obstetrics. 1992;**174**:7-10

[5] Lortat-Jacob JL, Robert HG, Henry C. Un cas d'hépatectomie droite réglée. Mémoires. Académie de Chirurgie. 1952; **78**:244-251

[6] Tung TT, Quang ND. L'hépatectomie réglée par ligature vasculaire intra-parenchymateuse. Presse Médicale. 1965;**73**:3015-3017

[7] Bismuth H, Castaing D, Garden OJ. Major hepatic resection under total vascular exclusion. Annals of Surgery. 1989;**210**:13-19

[8] Bismuth H, Houssin D, Ornowski J, Meriggi F. Liver resection in cirrhotic patients: A western experience. World Journal of Surgery. 1986;**10**:311-317

[9] Azoulay D, Raccuia JS, Castaing D, Bismuth H. Right portal vein embolization in preparation for major hepatic resection. Journal of the American College of Surgeons. 1995;**181**: 267-269

[10] Bismuth H, Castaing D. Echographie per-opératoire du foie et des voies biliaires. Paris: Flammarion Médecine-Sciences Ed; 1985

[11] Castaing D, Garden J, Bismuth H. Segmental liver resection using ultrasound-guided selective portal venous occlusion. Annals of Surgery. 1989;**210**:20-23

[12] Shimamura Y, Gunven P, Takenaka Y, Shimizu H, Akimoto H, Shima Y, et al. Selective portal branch occlusion by balloon catheter during liver resection. Surgery. 1986;**100**:938-941

[13] Gotoh M, Monden M, Sakon M, Kanai T, Umeshita K, Nagano H, et al. Hilar lobar vascular occlusion for hepatic resection. Journal of the American College of Surgeons. 1994; **178**:6-10

[14] Hannoun L, Vaillant JC, Borie D, Delva E. Techniques de l'exclusion vasculaire du foie et des hépatectomies extrêmes (chirurgie «ex situ-ex vivo» et «in situ-ex vivo» du foie). Encycl méd.-Chir., Techniques Chirurgicales - Appareil Digestif. Vol. 40. Paris: Editions Techniques Ed; 1994. pp. 766-782

[15] Belghiti J, Guevara OA, Noun R, Saldinger PF, Kianmanesh R. Liver hanging Manoeuvre : A safe approach to right hepatectomy without liver mobilization. Journal of the American College of Surgeons. 2001;**193**:109-111

[16] Ogata S, Belghiti J, Varma D, Sommacale D, Maeda A, Dondero F, et al. Two hundred hanging manoeuvres for major hepatectomy: A single-centre experience. Annals of Surgery. 2007; **245**:31-35

[17] Hirai I, Murakami G, Kimura W, Kanamura T, Sato I. How should we treat short hepatic veins and paracaval branches in anterior hepatectomy. Clinical Anatomy. 2003;**16**(3):224-232

Chapter 6

Liver Transplantation in China

Yingzi Ming, Quan Zhuang, Baoren Tu, Gangcheng Kong, Hao Li, Ying Niu, Bo Peng, Junhui Li, Meng Yu and Min Yang

Abstract

Liver transplantation has been developed in Mainland China for about 40 years, from clinical trials to maturity. Its number has become the second in the world, its quality is also in line with the international level, and the source of donors has gradually transitioned to donation after citizen's death (DCD). This chapter is aimed to elaborate the liver transplant work in China from the history and current status of liver transplantation, the main operating methods, major indications, donor maintenance and donor quality assessment, postoperative major complications, and application of immunosuppressive agents to the postoperative follow-up. Liver transplantation is a meaningful and challenging work currently in China; all the Chinese transplant surgeons and scholars are devoting themselves to this work in order to give more effective help to the patients.

Keywords: liver transplantation, Mainland China, DCD, piggyback liver transplantation, donor quality assessment, liver transplant indications, HBV, liver transplant complications, immunosuppressant, follow-up

1. The developing history and current status of liver transplantation in China

Since the first clinical trial of liver transplantation in Mainland China in 1977, it has been more than 40 years. During this period, China's liver transplantation has experienced ups and downs and finally developed from immature to mature. Liver transplantation has been recognized as the only effective treatment for various end-stage liver diseases. The number of liver transplant cases in China ranks second in the world, ranking behind the United States. Its rapid development has attracted the attention of the world, and it has also exposed many problems that need to be solved [1].

The development of liver transplantation in China has gone through the following stages:

(1) The initial trial stage (1977–1983). In 1977, Shanghai Ruijin Hospital and Wuhan Tongji Hospital started the clinical liver transplantation in China. From 1977 to 1983, 57 liver transplants were carried out nationwide, but because the liver transplantation indications at that time were mainly advanced primary liver cancer, the curative effect was poor, and most patients died 3 months after surgery. Ten years later (1983–1993), China's liver transplantation was basically at a standstill.

(2) Re-development stage (1993–1997). With the continuous entry of new immunosuppressants into China, the continuous improvement of surgical

techniques and perioperative management, and the continuous strengthening of international exchanges and cooperation, China's liver transplantation finally re-emerged in the 1990s.

(3) Rapid development stage (1997–2005). This is the main stage of liver transplantation development in China, and the main performance is as follows: (1) the number of liver transplants in mainland China has increased year by year. From 16 cases in 1997 to 100 cases in 1999, there were 200 cases of liver transplantation in 2000. By 2005, 3300 cases of liver transplantation were implemented. (2) The units and regions for liver transplantation have also increased year by year. More than 300 hospitals across the country have carried out liver transplantation. (3) Liver transplantation is diversified, from traditional classic liver transplantation to piggyback liver transplantation, ectopic liver transplantation, partial liver transplantation, split liver transplantation, and living donor liver transplantation. (4) The postoperative management level is continuously improved, the application of immunosuppressive agents is more individualized and diverse, and the survival rate of recipients is significantly improved. The 1-year survival rate after liver transplantation was 80.5%, and the 5-year survival rate was 65.9%. Liver transplantation technology and clinical efficacy are close to international standards [2]. In 2006, the Ministry of Health conducted an access work for organ transplant medical institutions, and China's liver transplantation entered the stage of clinical normative development. Liver transplantation is gradually incorporated into the legal management. The medical institutions that are admitted are mainly strong medical institutions that have mature liver transplantation technology and talented echelons. Taking the service area and scope into account, the admitted liver transplant medical institutions are mainly concentrated in the affiliated hospitals of the provincial capital universities in the big cities, which further guarantee the quality, safety, and management of transplants [3]. In 2007, China's first "Human Organ Transplantation Regulations" was officially implemented, and the Ministry of Health also issued relevant supporting regulations, marking a crucial step in the legalization and standardization of China's organ transplantation [4]. In February 2005, the China Liver Transplant Registration Network was established. The system was supported by the University of Hong Kong with the support of the Ministry of Health. In May 2008, the China Liver Transplant Registration Network was officially authorized by the Ministry of Health to further cover the 80 admitted liver transplantation centers [5]. China Liver Transplant Registration Network has been upgraded from scientific voluntary registration to administrative mandatory registration, becoming the standardized management system for liver transplantation in China. China Liver Transplant Network has collected more than 12,000 cases of domestic liver transplant patients. By the end of 2008, China had implemented 14,600 liver transplants. By August 10, 2009, China had implemented 16,158 liver transplants until July 22, 2010. The Chinese transplant network registered 18,180 liver transplants [6].

(4) DCD (organ donation after citizen's death) Liver transplantation stage (2010–present) in 2010. China gradually began trial of DCD for liver transplantation, with 11 provinces including Zhejiang, Yunnan, Hubei, and Hunan as the first batch of pilots. The DCD was vigorously promoted and achieved good results. Summary after the completion of the pilot work: as of July 1, 2013, a total of 906 DCD donors donated nationwide, and 2469 organs were donated, including 746 livers. The above data show that although the Chinese DCD work

started late, in the future it is the most potential source of organs [7]. Under the vigorous promotion of the Ministry of Health and the Red Cross Society, DCD work began to be promoted nationwide in 2012, and the construction of relevant laws and regulations also steadily advanced. In October 2012, in order to better implement the "Human Organ Transplant Regulations" and actively promote the Chinese organ donation work, the Ministry of Health formulated the "Management Methods for the Acquisition and Distribution of Human Organs in China" and established the "China Organ transplant response system" (OTRS). Through the application of this system, we wish to improve the matching degree of organs, reduce or prevent waste of resources, strive to achieve the traceability of each distributed organ, and eliminate the interference of human and subjective factors to ensure the principle of "fairness, openness, and justice" [8]. In 2010, DCD liver transplantation accounted for only 1.38% of the total, and in 2013, it has increased significantly to 26.02% [9], and by 2015, it has exceeded 80% [10]. China has completely banned the use of organs in the judicial channel since 2015. DCD donor China has become the main source of donors for organ transplantation in China. In 2017, 4732 cases of liver transplantation were performed in China, including 4138 cases of DCD liver transplantation, which was 26.43% higher than that of 2016 (3273 cases). The data show that the survival rates of liver transplantation in China at 1, 3, and 5 years are 84, 75, and 71%, respectively. The Chinese organ transplantation has entered the DCD era [11].

Although China's organ transplants have developed rapidly, they have also achieved many achievements and showed the characteristics of China, but they also exposed some problems.

(1) Problems faced by liver transplantation for liver cancer.

China is a big country with hepatitis B. The HBV carrying rate is about 10% in the national population. As the terminal end of the development chain of hepatitis-cirrhosis-hepatocarcinoma, the high incidence of liver cancer in China is inevitable. China's liver cancer patients account for more than half of the world's liver cancer patients, and 318,000 new liver cancer patients occur in China each year. With the continuous improvement of the medical insurance system, China has the world's largest transplant recipient group, liver cancer liver transplantation once accounted for about 44% of China's total liver transplant [5]. It is urgent to formulate the staging criteria and surgical adaptation of liver cancer liver transplantation in accordance with China's national conditions as soon as possible. At the same time, how to combine immunosuppressive agents with antiliver disease and antihepatitis virus treatment is the main problem faced by Chinese transplant experts [12].

(2) Problems faced by the DCD era.

The development of DCD donors has effectively alleviated the problem of donor shortages in China, and has also led to the complete abolition of judicial source donors. However, the current organ donation rate in China is still very low. In 2010, it was only 0.03 cases/million population. In 2015, it was 2.03 cases/million population, and in 2016, it was 2.98 cases/million population [13]. Although the growth is relatively fast, there is still a huge growth potential. This requires all levels of government in China to increase the propaganda of donations, and at the same time increase the staff of organ donation to find and report the information of potential donors in a timely manner. At the same time, a complete organ donation process must be developed to ensure the smooth implementation of the donation.

(3) Basic and clinical research related to transplantation needs to be strengthened.

Organ transplantation is a multidisciplinary and interdisciplinary profession. Only by strengthening relevant basic and clinical research, can we better protect organ quality and provide better postoperative management and monitoring of patients [14].

(4) The relevant laws and regulations on transplantation have yet to be perfected.

The current regulations on organ transplantation in China are mainly based on "the Interim Provisions on the Clinical Application Management of Human Organs Technology" issued in July 2006 and the "Human Organ Transplantation Regulations" promulgated by the State Council in March 2017. However, with the development of transplantation and the advent of the DCD era, more completed legal and ethical systems and management norms are needed to provide legal protection and policy support for the healthy and orderly development of organ transplantation in China.

China's clinical liver transplantation has entered a critical period of simultaneous hopes and challenges, and Chinese liver transplant experts are constantly working hard to make liver transplantation a better way for patients with liver disease.

2. Quality assessment of liver grafts

In China, liver grafts used for transplantation are mainly from DCD (organ donation after citizen's death), which includes DBD, DCD, DBCD, and living related donor. Here, we discuss the quality assessment of liver grafts from DCD. The quality of transplant liver is an important factor affecting the short-term and long-term effects of transplantation. Donated liver assessment mainly includes donor's general information, medical history, general condition and intervention, laboratory results, etc. and specific items are listed in **Table 1** [15]. Every case is evaluated dynamically, including at least one preliminary evaluation and final assessment prior to liver harvest. Donor age, hepatic steatosis, warm and cold ischemia time, the risk of infection and tumor, hypernatremia, etc. are risk factors affecting the quality of liver grafts.

2.1 Donor age

It is generally believed that elderly donors often have higher opportunity of getting arteriosclerosis, hepatic steatosis, and tumor, which are risk factors affecting the quality of liver. Therefore, age is an important factor in the evaluation of liver grafts, and usually, donor age > 50 years is considered a contraindication to the use for transplantation. However, as the progression of liver transplantation and the relatively expanded need for liver grafts, liver grafts from these elderly donors can also be used with rigorous assessment, especially in the case of ensuring a short warm and cold ischemia time [16–18].

2.2 Hepatic steatosis

Hepatic steatosis is an important factor affecting liver function after transplantation; hence, the classification and the grading of hepatic steatosis are extremely

Category	Item	Category	Item
General information of donor	Gender	Laboratory tests	Blood routine
	Age		Urine routine
	Blood type		Fecal routine
	Height		Liver function
	BMI		Blood lipids
Medical history	Primary disease (cause of death)		Blood sugar
	ICU stay days		Blood electrolytes
	Past history		Coagulation function
	Family history		HIV
General condition and intervention	Vital signs		Hepatitis virus
	Urine volume		Syphilis tests
	Mechanical ventilation		Tumor markers
	Vasoactive drugs and other related drugs		Infection-related indicators
Other	Judgment during harvesting operation		
	Warm and cold ischemia time		
	Pretransplant biopsies of livers		

Table 1.
Assessment content of liver grafts.

pivotal. According to the histology classification, hepatic steatosis is mainly divided into macrovesicular steatosis, which is considered to be a more dangerous one, and microvesicular steatosis, which is generally regarded as being reversible. For microvesicular steatosis liver grafts, even though the lesion is severe, they can still be used. For macrovesicular steatosis liver grafts, if the lesion is more than 50%, it is considered to be a taboo for transplantation [19, 20]. At present, the methods for evaluating fatty liver graft mainly relies on the judgment of organ harvesting surgeon, and rapid frozen biopsy of liver grafts [21, 22]. The research toward the use of imaging methods such as ultrasound, CT, MRI, and metabonomics in the assessment of liver steatosis is launched and their efficiency still need to be verified [23].

2.3 Warm and cold ischemia injury

Warm ischemic injury caused by hypotensive and hypoxic perfusion process is one of the most important features of liver grafts. Long-term ischemia can increase the risk of primary nonfunction and biliary complications; thus, the time of warm ischemia is an important factor in evaluating the quality of liver. In addition, cold ischemia time > 8 hours is also a risk factor of liver transplantation. It has been reported that the incidence of liver failure after transplantation increases by 8% for every 1 hour after cold ischemia time > 6 hours. Therefore, during the process of liver acquisition, in order to improve the quality of grafts, the operation and transportation time should be shortened as much as possible [18].

2.4 Hepatitis virus infection

It is mainly hepatitis B virus prevailing in China. The main route of HBV infection in liver transplant recipients is through liver grafts. Liver graft from the donor who is in active period of hepatitis virus infection or has developed hepatitis virus-related liver fibrosis should not be used. For HBV-positive grafts, they can still be used to recipients who are selected rationally, get prophylactic antiviral therapy and the treatment of HBV immunoglobulin [18, 19]. HCV infection is not common in China. HCV-positive liver grafts can be used to recipients who need transplantation urgently, and they need anti-HCV therapy after surgery.

2.5 Tumor

For donors who have malignant tumors or tumor history, whether the liver can be used for transplantation remains controversial, and the transfer risk of tumor cannot be properly assessed. It is generally believed that the incidence of donor-related tumor and the resulting mortality are very low. However, the current view is that the liver from donors who have malignant tumor history should be selected carefully because some malignant tumors have unpredictable possibilities of recurrence and metastasis [19].

2.6 Hypernatremia

Hypernatremia (serum sodium >155 mmol/L) in donors is an important factor affecting the prognosis of liver transplantation. Studies have shown that hypernatremia affects the function of transplant organs and increases the risk of liver failure after transplantation, whose mechanism may be related to cell swelling, increased osmotic pressure, and reperfusion injury caused by hypernatremia. This adverse effect can be reduced by effectively correcting the blood sodium concentration [18].

2.7 Liver preservation

The effect of liver preservation affects the quality of grafts. At present, there are two methods of liver storage, which are static cold storage (SCS) and mechanical perfusion (MP). SCS is the most widely used method, and UW liquid, HTK liquid and Celsior liquid are the most popular preservation liquids. The ideal time for cold storage is less than 8 hours, and in clinical practice, the preservation time generally does not exceed 12–15 hours. MP can continuously infuse the organ's intrinsic vascular system to deliver nutrient, achieve organ preservation, and repair simultaneously, having great value in prolonging the time of liver preservation and improving organ quality. Besides, MP can monitor liver function, bile secretion and other indicators dynamically during storage and transportation, and evaluate the quality of donated liver, showing important clinical application prospects [24, 25].

3. Donor liver procurement and benchwork surgery

3.1 Donor liver procurement

Since there is still no law about brain death, at the present stage in China, the sources of liver are DCD and living-related donation. Here, we only talk about the DCD donor liver procurement.

It is recommended in most centers the "rapid cold perfusion and en-bloc liver-kidney procurement" technique [26]. Core temperature of the liver can be decreased rapidly to 0–4°C by double perfusion from the hepatic artery (aortic cannulation) and the portal vein (superior mesenteric vein cannulation). This technique also prevents accidental injuries to the hepatic hilar structures.

Following administration of 30,000 IU or 300 IU/Kg of heparin, expeditious access to the abdominal cavity is obtained through a midline incision from the xiphoid to the pubic symphysis. The abdominal aorta and inferior vena cava (IVC) are dissected and cannulated, and the cold flush (0–4°C normal saline) is initiated immediately. Superior mesenteric vein is isolated and cannulated at the root of small bowel mesentery followed with perfusion. Ice and slush are packed around the liver and kidneys, and subsequent dissection is carried out after completion of cold perfusion (**Figure 1**).

The liver is mobilized by dividing the round ligament, falciform, left triangular, and gastrohepatic ligaments. The hepatoduodenal ligament, posterior peritoneum nearby and the adhesions between the head of pancreas and duodenum are dissected with modified Kocher maneuver; the common bile duct is exposed and transected at the inferior margin of pancreas. The whole colon, stomach, and duodenum are isolated successively; then the bilateral peritoneum are cut open and the peritoneal attachments in the retroperitoneal space are divided until the spine. The ureters are isolated and transected at the common iliac artery level. After the procedure, only the liver, spleen, kidneys, and most part of pancreas are still left in the abdominal cavity. The pericardium and diaphragm are incised bilaterally: on the left, extending to the esophagus, and on the right, extending posterior the right lobe of the liver, adrenal gland, and IVC. The thoracic aorta and IVC are transected

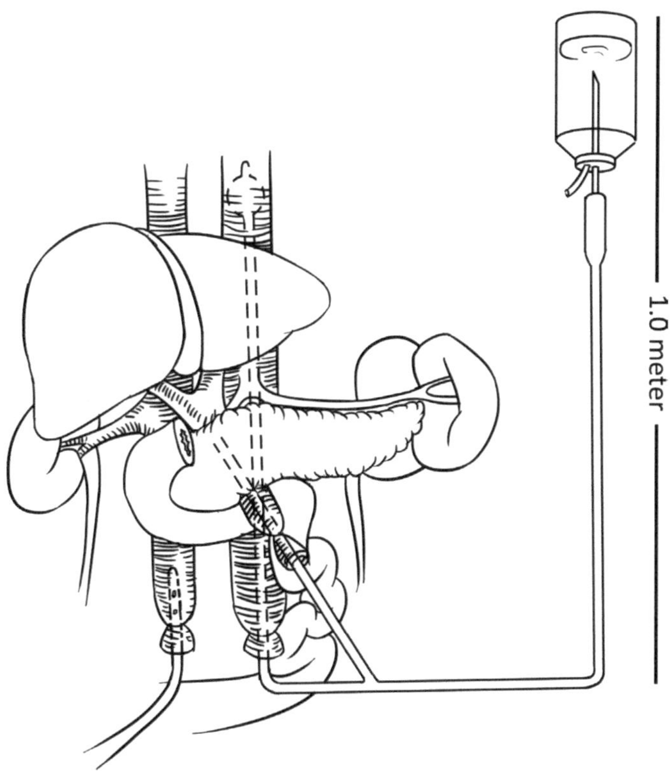

Figure 1.
The intubation perfusion of aorta and portal vein.

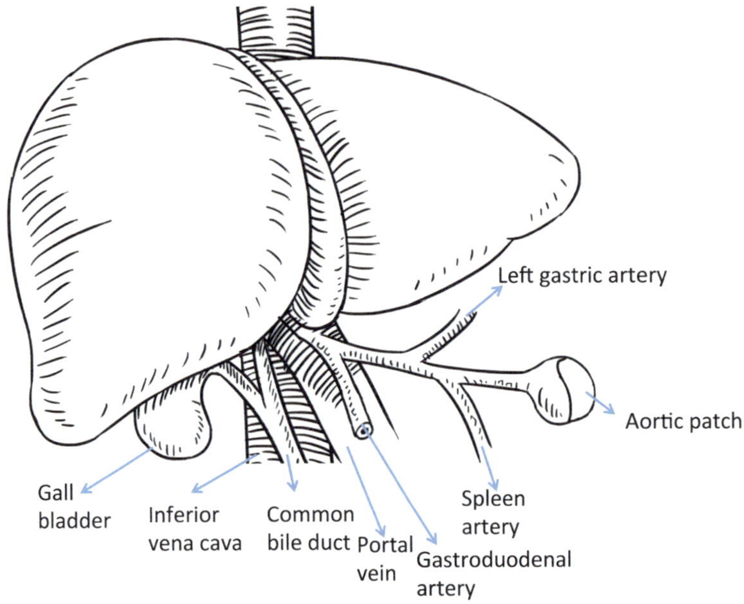

Figure 2.
The trimmed and shaped donor liver.

and the adhesions with the spine are divided until the common iliac artery level. The en-bloc liver-kidney-spleen organs cluster can be harvested with the aorta and IVC transection just below the cannulas.

Once the multiple-organs cluster is taken out, it must be put into the sterile basin filled with 0–4°C organ preservation solution (usually UW solution) immediately. Additional perfusion usually is needed in order to eliminate the residual blood and sustain the low core temperature of the organs. The posterior wall of the aorta is longitudinal cut out, and the origins of celiac truck, superior mesenteric artery (SMA) and bilateral kidney arteries are exposed. The adhesions between the right kidney, adrenal gland, and the hepatic right lobe are divided until the inferior IVC exposed. IVC is transected just above the kidney veins level, and aorta is transected below the origin of SMA level; the liver and kidneys are separated and packaged respectively.

3.2 Bench surgery

The aim of bench surgery is to remove the unnecessary tissues attached to the liver and trim the main vessels and bile duct for a convenient anastomosis. The bench should be set up with a suitable sized bowl in which the graft is kept in sterile slush ice and UW at 4°C for the duration of the procedure to avoid rewarming.

Firstly, the diaphragm and remaining cardiac muscle are removed from the bare area of the liver and the vena cava. Then, the supra- and intrahepatic vena cava are skeletonized and all small branches are ligated with silk. The adrenal vein and the phrenic veins are tied or over sewn to prevent bleeding upon recirculation.

The skeletonization of the hepatic artery is the most critical step in the bench surgery procedure. The dissection starts from the aorta and ends until the gastro duodenal artery (GDA) in order not to injure the hepatic lobar vessels. Care is taken to identify any aberrant arterial anatomy, which can be present in up to 20% of the population [27]. So, every artery and its branches should be isolated until it is identified that not entering the liver. The most common two variants are a replaced right hepatic artery emanating from superior mesenteric artery or a replaced left hepatic artery originating from the left gastric artery. Often the aberrant liver arteries need to be reconstructed for anastomosis.

The portal vein is skeletonized up to 1–2 cm below the bifurcation point. Surrounding lymphatic tissue is removed, and care is taken not to injure the hepatic artery or bile duct.

The pancreas tissues around the lower segment of the common bile duct are removed. Do not dissect excessively the tissues between the bile duct and the hepatic artery in order to preserve the blood supply of the bile duct.

A perfusion-giving set with cold UW should be set up to perfuse the liver and also to check the integrity of the portal vein and arterial tree, once the graft has been prepared for implantation (**Figure 2**).

4. Surgical methods of recipient liver transplantation

Surgical methods of recipient liver transplantation include two main categories: orthotopic liver transplantation and ectopic liver transplantation [28]. At present, transplant centers in China basically use orthotopic liver transplantation. Orthotopic liver transplantation is divided into classic orthotopic liver transplantation, piggy-back orthotopic liver transplantation, reduced-size liver transplantation, split liver transplantation, and auxiliary liver transplantation according to different surgical methods. The above procedures are applied in the Chinese transplant centers.

4.1 Classical orthotopic liver transplantation

4.1.1 Diseased liver resection

A curved cut under the regular costal edge or "Mercedes-Benz" logo shape incision has been made firstly, then dissecting the first hepatic portal dissecting the hepatic artery, separating the common bile duct, and finally separating the portal vein [29]. The inferior vena cava is then exposed. The posterior inferior vena cava can be quickly and safely separated from the posterior peritoneum [30].

4.1.2 Extracorporeal portal

The nonhepatic venous bypass technique can reduce the congestion of the portal system and can solve the problem of blood return in the intestine and inferior vena cava during the nonhepatic period [31, 32]. As the surgical techniques become more and more skilled, the anastomosis time is shortened. At present, most transplant centers in China have adopted nontransfer liver transplantation technology [33]. However, for patients with severe hepatorenal syndrome, gastrointestinal bleeding, and cardiac insufficiency before surgery, extracorporeal portal bypass technology will still benefit.

4.1.3 Graft implantation

The portal vein and two inferior vena cava were clamped in turn, to avoid vascular torsion, and the blood vessels were cut off near the liver to remove the diseased liver. The suprahepatic inferior vena cava the infrahepatic inferior vena cava and the portal vein were sequentially anastomosed with 3-0, 4-0, and 5-0 Prolene sutures. The anastomosis was performed by two-point continuous valgus suture. Precautions of inferior vena cava anastomosis: A. The inferior vena cava of the recipient and the donor cannot be kept too long or too short; otherwise, the inferior vena cava will be folded or stretched, and the inferior vena cava hypertension or bleeding will be caused. B. The recipient's suprahepatic inferior vena cava cannot be reversed; otherwise, it will cause poor blood flow in the inferior vena cava. C. The suture cannot be pulled too tightly to avoid damage to the intima form artificial stenosis, and even lead to Budd-Chiari syndrome. Precautions of hepatic portal vein anastomosis: A. Donor and recipient's portal vein should be kept proper. B. The difference between the size of the portal vein of the donor and the recipient should not be too large, otherwise. C. The tension of the anastomosis needs to be appropriate. When the suture is completed, the "widening factor" of the portal vein should also be retained. The transplanted liver blood flow is then opened. The hepatic artery was reconstructed with a 7-0 Prolene suture, and the hepatic artery was opened. Successful hepatic artery reconstruction is critical to the function of the transplanted liver and the influence of bile duct. There is a variety of suturing methods: A. Separate the hepatic artery, the gastro duodenal artery and the common hepatic artery, and the three confluences were trimmed as a hornline, which was anastomosed with the donor's common hepatic artery. B. When the gastroduodenal artery is relatively large, the donor's celiac trunk artery can be anastomosed at the junction of the recipient's gastroduodenal artery and the proper hepatic artery. C. If there is an anatomic abnormality in the hepatic artery of the donor, the hepatic artery should be trimmed, shaped, and then anastomosed with the recipient's hepatic artery. D. When the recipient's hepatic artery has an anatomic abnormality, the donor's celiac trunk artery can be directly anastomosed to the abdominal aorta above the recipient's celiac trunk artery. Finally, the bile duct was reconstructed with a 6-0 or 7-0 Prolene suture. T tube is drawn through the recipient's common bile duct. If the recipient's common bile duct is very small, it is recommended to perform bile duct jejunum Roux-en-Y anastomosis. The graft gallbladder was then removed [34–36] (**Figure 3**).

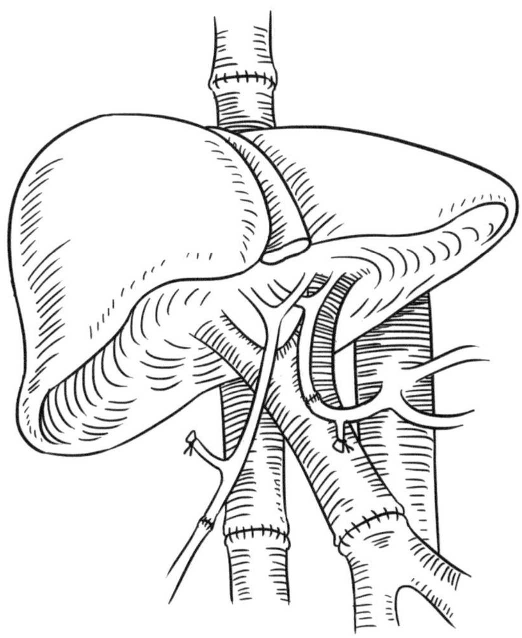

Figure 3.
The classical orthotopic liver transplantation.

4.2 Piggyback liver transplantation

Piggyback liver transplantation, different from the classical liver transplantation, is that the infrahepatic inferior vena cava is not necessary to be anastomosed, which thereby is clamped, and the suprahepatic inferior vena cava of the donor liver is anastomosed directly to the recipient's hepatic vein or laterally to the recipient's inferior vena cava [37, 38]. This procedure simplifies the operation of donor liver implantation, and only partially blocks the inferior vena cava during operation. It has little effect on hemodynamics in patients in nonhepatic phase, does not require venous bypass, and has less renal damage. However, this traditional piggyback liver transplantation procedure has a problem that the graft liver would swing in the abdominal cavity and cause vascular torsion, and the circulation return will be affected. At present, the modified piggyback procedure used in most mature transplant centers in China is below: inferior vena cava (VC) shaping: (1) recipient VC: according to the patient's hepatic vein anatomy, the hepatic veins (left, middle and right) are split from the middle and trimmed into a continuous opening, and the front wall of inferior vena cava is also trimmed longitudinally, and all these together form an inverted triangular incision. (2) Donor VC: the posterior wall of the donor superior inferior vena cava was cut longitudinally with the two up angers of hepatic superior VC, also trimmed into an inverted triangular incision. Finally, these two inverted triangular incisions are anastomosed (**Figure 4**). The main purpose of this piggyback procedure is to enlarge the anastomosis of the outflow tract, avoid the anastomotic torsion, and reduce the incidence of postoperative outflow obstruction [39, 40].

4.3 Reduced-size liver transplantation and split liver transplantation

In our clinical work, the whole liver transplantation cannot meet the needs of liver transplantation in children and some small-weight adults, because these patients cannot accommodate the large-size liver in the abdominal cavity, which is why the reduced-size liver transplantation came into being [41]. Reduced-size liver transplantation actually includes reduced-size cadaveric liver transplantation, split liver transplantation, and partial living liver transplantation. By 2010, 86 transplant centers in 30 provinces of Mainland China had undergone reduced-size liver transplantation. The donor liver for children with reduced-size liver transplantation

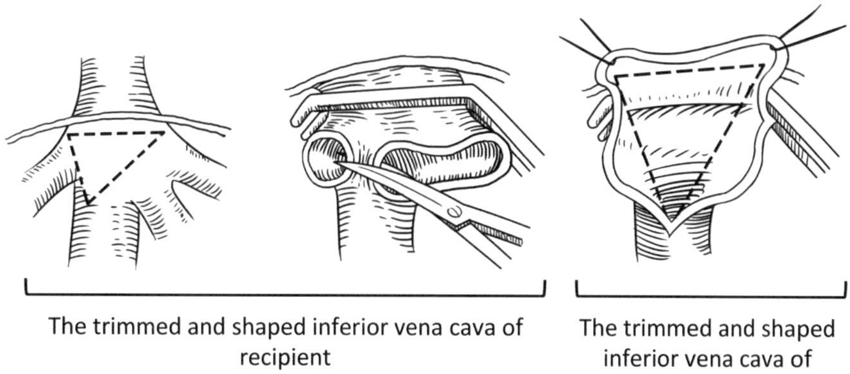

Figure 4.
The two "inverted triangular" incisions of donor and recipient's inferior CV.

is mainly the left liver. Split liver transplantation refers to the separation of an adult cadaveric donor liver into two transplanted livers with independent structures and functions by two-way technique, which is transplanted to two recipients. The conventional method is to detach the liver along the Cantlie line and obtain the intact right and left hepatic livers, respectively [42, 43].

4.4 Auxiliary liver transplantation

Auxiliary liver transplantation refers to retaining the recipient's liver or part of the liver, implanting the donor's whole liver or part of the liver into the recipient, so that patients with liver failure can receive life support or compensate for the metabolism, detoxification, and other functions of the original liver deficiency [44]. It is divided into auxiliary ectopic liver transplantation and auxiliary orthotopic liver transplantation. The auxiliary liver transplantation has the following advantages: (1) patients with acute liver failure can pass the dangerous period, and (2) for congenital metabolic liver disease, implantation of a small amount of liver can meet the patient's metabolic needs, (3) under surgical trauma, the recipient has no nonhepatic period, (4) the required liver volume is small, increase the donor liver source, and (5) for some patients within inability to tolerate the orthotopic whole liver transplantation, auxiliary liver transplantation should be performed first, and then the orthotopic liver transplantation should be considered after the recovery of the body function.

4.5 Living donor liver transplantation

Living donor liver transplantation has developed rapidly due to the severe lack of cadaver donor livers. In early years, the left half liver was used as the donor liver for living donor liver transplantation between adults, but for large-size recipients, the left half liver could not meet the demand of the recipient, so the right half liver was gradually used as the donor liver. The procedure of living donor liver transplantation is basically the same as that of orthotopic liver transplantation, but there are many differences in the reconstruction of hepatic vein, portal vein, hepatic artery, and bile duct.

4.5.1 Hepatic vein reconstruction

In living donor liver transplantation, the right half liver as donor liver is divided into two types, including the hepatic middle vein and not including the hepatic middle vein. Whether the branches of the hepatic middle vein in hepatic segment V and VIII should be reconstructed in living donor liver transplantation of right half liver is controversial. Different liver transplantation centers have proposed different reconstruction criteria.

In the literature, B ultrasonography was used to assess congestion in the right half liver donation after temporary occlusion of the hepatic artery and the hepatic middle vein. Criteria for reconstruction of hepatic middle vein include: (1) after removing the area of the congestion, the remaining transplanted liver volume was less than 40% of recipient's standard liver volume. (2) When hepatic artery and hepatic middle vein branches are blocked, the area of the donor liver congestion is more than half of the area of the right anterior lobe. (3) Noncongestive graft-to-recipient weight ratio (ncGRWR) $< 0.65\%$.

The diameter of the branches of the hepatic middle vein is also one of the criteria for reconstruction. The diameter of the branch of the hepatic middle vein in hepatic segments V and VIII was more than 7 mm, which was considered as the boundary of whether to reconstruct the branch of the hepatic middle vein. Kim et al. suggested that when the hepatic middle vein branches of segments V and VIII were larger than 5 mm in diameter, the hepatic middle vein branches needed to be reconstructed, and they tried to make the area of congestion less than 10% of the total graft volume [45].

In living liver transplantation without hepatic middle vein, the grafts used for reconstruction of hepatic middle vein include the recipient's own great saphenous vein, superficial femoral vein, umbilical vein, portal vein, artificial blood vessel, iliac vein or iliac artery cryopreserved from allogeneic tissue, and also venous patch to reconstruct the branch of hepatic umbilical vein. Liver transplantation center of the first Hospital of Zhejiang University carried out a preliminary study on 131 cases of living right donor liver transplantation without hepatic middle vein. The graft vessels were reconstructed by autologous portal vein, hepatic vein, great saphenous vein, or cryopreserved iliac artery to reconstruct the right hepatic vein branches V and VIII without hepatic middle vein [5].

4.5.2 Portal vein construction

After the portal veins of donor liver and recipient were in line with their caliber and length, they were performed with an end-to-end anastomosis. When the recipient of living donor liver transplantation has portal vein sclerosis or narrow problems, we anastomose the donor portal vein directly to the confluence of the recipient's splenic vein and superior mesenteric vein. If the donor portal vein does not have enough length, portal vein transplantation can be performed.

4.5.3 Hepatic artery reconstruction

The reconstruction of hepatic artery in living donor liver transplantation is directly related to the success or failure of transplantation. The diameter of donor hepatic artery is only 2–3 mm. Arterial anastomosis under direct vision has been a difficult problem for many surgeons. Until the application of microsurgical vascular anastomosis under microscope, the incidence of hepatic artery thrombosis decreased from 25 to 0–3.8%. However, this technique is difficult to master and is influenced by arterial variations, donor-recipient caliber matching, and recipient hemodynamics. Therefore, it is important to establish a stable microsurgical team and mature arterial anastomosis methods in various transplantation centers.

4.5.4 Bile duct reconstruction

(1) Bile duct shaping: within 3 mm, the combination of adjacent hepatic duct opening can be considered.

(2) The principle of one-time suture insertion: in the so-called one-time suture process, the noninvasive suture needle from the recipient of the bile duct to the donor of the hepatic duct needle, must be completed at one time

(3) The basic bile duct end to end anastomosis technique: the posterior wall is continuously sutured, and the anterior wall is discontinuously sutured.

With the improvement of liver transplantation anesthesia, surgical techniques and perioperative management, the efficacy and survival rate of liver transplant patients have been significantly improved. With the accumulation of surgical experience, we need promotion of our surgical techniques. However, in view of the current situation of organ shortage in China, how to choose the most suitable liver transplantation for different indications, preoperative status, and physiological and anatomical features still needs to continuously explore and summarize the experience.

5. Complications after liver transplantation

5.1 Early complications after liver transplantation

5.1.1 Postliver transplant hemorrhage

Intraabdominal hemorrhage postliver transplantation is an early serious complication, and continues to be a prognostic factor for transplant success. Statistically, intraabdominal hemorrhage postliver transplantation occurs in 5–21% of recipients [46], while incidence rate of this complication in China is 5–15.3% [47, 48]. Reasons for intraabdominal bleeding after liver transplantation include coagulopathy, portal hypertension, massive transfusion of stored blood, primary graft non-function/poor graft function, anastomotic leakage, as well as blood vessel damage by abdominal infection. Coagulopathy is one of the most important risk factors for postoperative early hemorrhage. Diffuse hemorrhage postreperfusion often occurs in recipients with coagulopathy, especially in those with poor liver function or lack of clotting factors. In addition, massive transfusion of stored blood leads to circulatory overload, abnormal coagulation and acid-base imbalance, resulted with aggravated hemorrhage symptoms. Surgical bleeding is related with operation of liver resection or graft harvesting. Furthermore, early hemorrhage may also occur as a result of blood vessel damage caused by anastomotic leakage or abdominal infection. Therefore, keeping normal coagulation function perioperatively, reducing bleeding and achieving effective hemostasis during operation, accurate anastomosis of blood vessels with vascular patency, as well as preventing and controlling infection, can contribute to prevention of this complication.

Therapeutically, correcting the clotting problem via giving blood products and coagulants is usually effective. However, patients with persistent hemodynamic instability, which indicates active hemorrhage, usually require emergency exploratory laparotomy for hemostasis.

5.1.2 Vascular complications

Vascular complications represent one of the most critical complications, and contribute to a major source of morbidity and mortality after liver transplantation. Vascular complications, including hepatic arterial complications, portal vein complications and vena cava complications, threaten outcomes for liver transplant recipients and graft survival. Among the vascular complications, hepatic arterial complications following liver transplantation are the most threatening conditions, including hepatic arterial thrombosis (HAT), hepatic artery stenosis, hepatic artery aneurysm, and hepatic artery rupture.

HAT is a life-threatening complication, as it interrupts blood supply of the allograft and induces early graft loss, long-term graft dysfunction, or recipient death. As the most common hepatic arterial complication, HAT occurs in 2–9% of adult transplants with a higher incidence in pediatric recipients [49, 50]. Risk factors for the development of HAT include technical imperfection with the anastomosis, dissection of the hepatic arterial wall, celiac stenosis or compression by median arcuate ligament, aberrant arterial anatomy, complex back-table arterial reconstruction of the allograft, as well as high-resistance microvascular arterial outflow mediated by rejection or severe ischemic-reperfusion injury. According to the time of onset, HAT is divided into early HAT and late HAT. Early HAT, diagnosed less than 4 weeks after liver transplantation, shows various clinical manifestations, ranging from fulminant hepatic failure, recurrent biliary sepsis, or delayed biliary leaks to an asymptomatic presentation with abnormal liver function. Compared with early HAT, clinical presentation of late HAT is relatively reduced, varied from increased serum transaminase level with or without cholestasis to liver abscess and biliary complications such as ischemic biliary lesions, cholangitis, bile duct stenosis, or necrosis. Early diagnosis with emergent surgical intervention is lifesaving and contributes to graft survival. Diagnosis of HAT depends on imaging examinations, while surgical exploration can confirm diagnosis. In clinical setting, arteriography is recognized as gold standard for diagnosis of HAT following liver transplantation. Patients with early HAT and fulminant hepatic failure require resuscitation, broad-spectrum antibiotics, artificial liver, and expeditious retransplantation.

Hepatic artery stenosis is one of the most common complications postliver transplantation, with incidence rate ranging from 4 to 11% [51, 52]. This stenosis most commonly occurs in anastomosis site or the kinking of reconstructed artery. Factors associated with hepatic artery stenosis include surgical injury, vasospasm, anastomotic stenosis, high-resistance hepatic artery blood flow mediated by rejection, and cold preservation injury. Clinical presentation varies from abnormal liver function to severe biliary complications. If unrecognized and managed appropriately, hepatic artery stenosis will lead to complete occlusion of hepatic artery or thrombosis, resulting in ischemic infarction and graft failure. Angiography is the gold standard for diagnosis of hepatic artery stenosis. Therapeutically, interventional vascular procedures are current major treatment.

Hepatic artery aneurysm and hepatic artery rapture are rare complications after liver transplantation, with an incidence of 0.3–1% [53, 54]. However, these complications can also threaten patients and grafts.

5.1.3 Biliary complications

The incidence of biliary complications has decreased dramatically because of advances in liver transplantation; however, biliary complication remains the most frequent complications postliver transplantation, with an incidence of 26.92–53.8% [55, 56]. Biliary complication is no longer a major cause of mortality in experienced liver transplantation center, as these complications can be recognized early and revive timely effective management. But biliary complication exhibits impact on patients' life quality, and sometimes it enables development of graft dysfunction. Therefore, biliary complication remains a challenging complication.

Biliary complications include bile leakage, anastomosis stenosis, bile duct ischemic injury, gall-stone formation, and sphincter dysfunction. Bile leakage, either anastomosis leakage or bile leakage after removal of T-tubes, usually occurs early postliver transplantation. Anastomosis stenosis is frequent. Endoscopic therapy and interventional radiology treatment are proven to be effective in treatment of anastomosis stenosis. Bile duct ischemic injury is a major cause of bile leakage, bile duct stenosis, or dilatation, followed by biliary sludge and cholelithiasis. Gallstone formation is mainly found in donor liver bile duct, but can also be observed in recipient's bile duct. Sphincter dysfunction is a complication hard to diagnose. Among the biliary complications after liver transplantation, bile duct ischemic injury is the most dangerous disease with high mortality. Patients with serious bile duct ischemic injury finally will need retransplantation. Surgical imperfection and bile duct ischemia are the major causes of biliary complication. Accurate bile duct anastomosis without distortion of the bile duct, proper use of T-tube, avoiding excessive trimming of vessels, and protecting blood supply of bile duct will promote reconstruction of bile duct and reduce bile duct complications after liver transplantation. Immunosuppressants can also contribute to this complication, such as CsA promotes cholestasis and gall-stone formation.

Clinical presentation of biliary complication varies. Patients with bile leakage usually have mild or moderate abdominal pain, with bile drained out from drainage tube or biliary spillage from umbilical incision. Symptoms of serious bile duct stenosis include jaundice in a short time. Early symptoms of patients with bile duct ischemic injury are atypical, sometimes similar to bile leakage, but late symptoms of bile duct ischemic injury like bile duct stenosis. Gallstones may occur secondary to bile duct stenosis, and patients with serious bile duct obstruction usually will have abdominal pain and jaundice.

With advances in imaging and endoscopic therapy, biliary complications can be diagnosed early and interventional treatment has become the first choice for patients with biliary complications after liver transplantation.

5.2 Late complications

With advances in transplant technique, liver transplant recipients achieve a longer life longevity and prolonged graft survival. Meanwhile, late complications postliver transplantation gradually become critical factors of their life quality and graft long-term survival.

5.2.1 Metabolic complications

5.2.1.1 De novo diabetes

De novo diabetes after liver transplantation is critical for outcomes of patients, correlated with a higher incidence of infection or cardiovascular diseases postliver transplantation. And it contributes to graft dysfunction and lower recipients' survival. According to definition of diabetes mellitus from WHO and ADA, de novo diabetes occurs in 9–63.3% patients with liver transplantation [57, 58]. Immunosuppressants, such as corticosteroid use and calcineurin inhibition, are risk factors for de novo diabetes. Appropriate use of immunosuppressant, including dose and duration, is of significance for preventing de novo diabetes postliver transplantation.

5.2.1.2 Hyperlipidemia

Hyperlipidemia is a common complication is solid organ transplantation, which can significantly promote incidence of chronic cardiac diseases in organ recipients. The incidence rate of hyperlipidemia in liver recipients is 45–66% [48, 58, 59]. Elevations of serum cholesterol and triglyceride are common consequences of use of immunosuppressants. Particularly, steroids and cyclosporine are closely associated with higher levels of cholesterols and triglyceride, while sirolimus exerts a stronger impact on triglyceride levels. Life style modifications with diet, exercise, and weight loss are preferred treatments. Besides, HMG-CoA reductase inhibition requires caution, as it may cause hepatotoxicity.

5.2.1.3 Hyperuricemia

Hyperuricemia is common in patients with liver transplantation, which usually occurs in 17–60 months postliver transplantation. The incidence rate of hyperuricemia in patients received liver transplantation is 14–47% [60, 61]. Mechanically, long-term use of calcineurin inhibitors leads to kidney injury and impairs the capability to clear uric acid, resulted with elevated uric acid levels or gout.

5.2.2 Biliary complications

Although huge advances have been made in liver transplantation, including biliary reconstruction, organ preservation and perioperative management, the incidence of biliary complications after liver transplantation remains high, up to 53.8% [56]. Biliary complications include biliary stenosis, bile leakage, ampulla dysfunction, biliary silt, and gallstone formation. However, biliary stenosis and gallstone formation are major late complications. As biliary reconstruction is recognized as Achilles' heel of liver transplantation, biliary reconstruction technique is strongly correlated with biliary complications. Besides, poor blood supply of hepatic artery and injury caused by donor liver harvest, cold preservation, or reperfusion. Furthermore, infection is also an important cause of biliary complication.

5.2.3 Recurrent disease

Recurrent liver diseases after liver transplantation is a common late complication, including hepatitis B, nonalcoholic fatty liver disease, autoimmune hepatitis, primary biliary cirrhosis as well as primary sclerosing cholangitis; however, the risk and timing of recurrent liver diseases are variable. Of note, recurrent hepatitis B virus (HBV) infection can be prevented in compliant patients with hepatitis B immunoglobulin and anti-HBV drugs. However, poor therapy compliance with irregular immunosuppressants application allows recurrence of HBV infection. In addition, recurrent autoimmune hepatitis or primary biliary cirrhosis rarely cause graft dysfunction or require retransplantation, though there are no proven effective therapies for the treatment of these late complications.

6. Indications for liver transplantation

Liver transplantation is an important option to treat the end-stage liver diseases and aims to prolong the life survival and to improve the quality of life for the patients. In principle, any acute or chronic liver disease, which has no other effective treatment or would cause the death of the patient in a short time, should be the indication to liver transplantation. With the increasing advance of liver transplantation, it can also be performed to improve the quality of life, although the primary liver disease might not be cured. The detail indications include the following:

(a) Acute liver failure: infections, drug- or toxin-induced liver injury, circulatory disturbance, etc.

(b) Liver cirrhosis: hepatitis cirrhosis, alcoholic cirrhosis, cholestatic cirrhosis, etc.

(c) Liver neoplasms: hepatocellular carcinoma, cholangiocarcinoma, etc.

(d) Metabolic disorders: Wilson disease, alpha-1 antitrypsin deficiency, hereditary tyrosinemia, glycogen storage disease, etc.

(e) Others: autoimmune hepatitis, polycystic liver, trauma, etc.

The contraindications, although decreasing with the development of liver transplantation, generally include the following:

(a) Malignancy outside of the liver and cannot be radical cured

(b) Uncontrolled sepsis

(c) Excessive drinking or drug abuse

(d) Severe cardiopulmonary, encephalic or renal complications

(e) Acquired immunodeficiency syndrome (AIDS)

(f) Persistent nonadherence with medical care

(g) Uncontrolled psychological or mental diseases

According to the China Liver Transplant Registry (CLTR), the most common disease leading to liver transplantation from DCD was liver neoplasms (42.98%), following by liver cirrhosis (41.05%) and acute liver failure (9.07%) from 2010 to 2017. The model for end-stage liver disease (MELD) or MELDNa score is applied to evaluate the status of the patients and to determine the priority of recipients and the allocation of organs by the CLTR.

6.1 Liver transplantation for hepatocellular carcinoma

It was estimated that more than 300,000 patients died of hepatocellular carcinoma (HCC) in China, which accounted for half of the total deaths all over the world [62]. The main reason was the high rate of hepatitis B virus (HBV) infection. In recent years, liver transplantation has become an effective treatment to HCC, in which the en bloc resection of the tumor can be achieved and the cirrhotic liver can be replaced. According to the CLTR, HCC was one of the most common causes leading to liver transplantation from DCD in China, with the 1- and 5-year survival rate of 82.77 and 59.18%, respectively (CLTR, 2010–2017). With the large number of practices, the Chinese experience was summarized.

6.1.1 Indications

The Milan criteria (a single lesion ≤5 cm, or up to three lesions, all ≤5 cm; no macrovascular invasion; no regional nodal or extrahepatic distant metastases) are the benchmark for selection of appropriate candidates for liver transplantation due to HCC. However, few patients in clinical practice could fully meet these strict criteria so that they might lose the opportunity of transplantation. Even expanded to the University of California at San Francisco (UCSF) criteria or Pittsburgh criteria, the number of candidates meeting the criteria is still limited in China. During the past decades, many Chinese scholars tried to expand the boundary of the indication, and concluded the criteria suitable for the Chinese situation.

(1) Hangzhou Criteria.

The Hangzhou Criteria were proposed by Prof. Shu-Sen Zheng, etc. in 2008 [63]. The criteria contained one of the two following items: (a) total tumor diameter ≤8 cm; (b) total tumor diameter > 8 cm, with histopathologic grade I or II and preoperative alpha fetoprotein (AFP) level ≤ 400 ng/mL, simultaneously.

Obviously, Hangzhou Criteria significantly expanded the candidate pool, and the reported 5-year survival rate was comparable to that of patients fulfilling Milan criteria (72.3 versus 78.3%, $P > 0.05$). More importantly, these criteria not only considered the tumor size, but also included the histopathologic grading and serum AFP level, which better reflected the biological characteristics of the tumor and predicted the prognosis. In Chinese guidelines of liver transplantation to HCC 2014, Hangzhou criteria were recommended [62].

(2) Shanghai Fudan Criteria.

Compared to Milan criteria, Shanghai Fudan Criteria expanded the indications on the tumor size: single lesion ≤9 cm in diameter, or no more than three lesions, the largest ≤5 cm, with a total tumor diameter ≤ 9 cm. There was no significant difference in 1, 2, 3-year survival rates and recurrence-free survival rates between Milan criteria and Shanghai Fudan Criteria [64].

6.1.2 Downgrade treatment of HCC before transplantation

The early diagnosis of HCC in China is limited so that a large number of patients are diagnosed with advanced HCC. Even if the expanded criteria were applied, many patients still lose the opportunity of transplantation. For patients without macrovascular invasion or extrahepatic distant metastases but beyond the current indications, downgrade treatments are proved effective to make part of the patients available to liver transplantation [65, 66]. The main downgrade treatments include transcatheter hepatic arterial chemoembolization (TACE), and local ablation therapy (radiofrequency ablation, microwave ablation, cryoablation and percutaneous ethanol injection) [62]. The combination of multiple therapies may achieve better efficacy.

6.1.3 Antivirus treatment

It was reported that over 90% of the HCC patients in China were related to the HBV infection. The high HBV load would increase the risk of tumor recurrence so that antivirus treatment is recommended pre-, intra- and posttransplantation. Before transplantation, the candidate should receive the nucleotide analogues (NAs) like entecavir and tenofovir as soon as possible to reduce the HBV load. During the nonhepatic phase in operation, the hepatitis B immunoglobulin (HBIG) is administered to block the viral transmission. After transplantation, the combination of NAs and low-dose of HBIG is recommended. HBV vaccines are given to some recipients posttransplantation, but the effects are still controversial.

6.1.4 Immunosuppression and prevention of tumor recurrence

The triple immunosuppressive regimens (CNI + MMF + corticosteroids) still consist the footstone of immunosuppression for HCC liver transplantation. Although CNI is reported as an independent risk factor for tumor recurrence, complete drug withdraw is not recommended. The mammalian target of rapamycin (mTOR) inhibitor like sirolimus or everolimus, which has the potential for the inhibition of tumor growth, has been applied with the induction of IL-2 receptor antagonist (IL-2RA) in some centers in China. What is advocated currently is the individualized regimen based on the individual's immune status. The main regimens used in clinic include the followings: (1) CNI + MMF + corticosteroids, (2) IL-2RA + sirolimus/everolimus + MMF + corticosteroids, and (3) IL-2RA + sirolimus/everolimus + MMF [62].

The recurrence of HCC is the main hinder for the long-term survival of these patients. Reportedly, the recurrence rate reached 20.0–57.8%; thus, it is critical to prevent the recurrence posttransplantation [67, 68]. The effective treatments include 131I-labeled metuximab, sorafenib, and chemotherapy. The choice depends on the morphological features, neoplasm staging, gene typing, histological grade, and biological characteristics of the tumor.

6.2 Liver transplantation for viral hepatitis

In China, viral hepatitis is mostly caused by HBV infection, and the prevalence of HCV is low. National Hepatitis Serum Epidemiology Survey [69, 70] showed that the HBsAg carrier rate in China's general population aged 1–59 years was 7.18%, while the anti-HCV prevalence rate was about 0.43% [71]. Based on this, there are about 93 million people with chronic HBV infection [72], and for HCV infection, this data are 5.6–10 million [73]. Patients with end-stage chronic hepatitis B have become the main population of liver transplant recipients in China. According to the China Liver Transplant Registry (CLTR) 2015 statistics, patients with viral hepatitis-associated liver disease accounted for 74.79%, and hepatitis B virus (HBV)-related liver disease patients accounted for 71.25%. Therefore, the following mainly describes the problems faced by liver transplantation in the treatment of hepatitis B virus-associated liver disease.

6.2.1 Indications

Similar to other indications for liver transplantation in chronic liver disease, liver transplantation should be considered when the following conditions occur:

(a) Patients undergoing systemic medical treatment, but the expected survival time is shorter than 2 years

(b) Recurrent esophageal varices bleeding after endoscopic treatment

(c) Refractory ascites

(d) Chronic hepatic encephalopathy

(e) Occasional bacterial peritonitis

(f) Liver cancer that occurs on the basis of hepatitis B

6.2.2 Prevention of hepatitis B virus recurrence after transplantation

The choice of patients with viral liver disease as recipients of liver transplantation was once controversial. The main reason is the high recurrence rate of viral hepatitis after transplantation. Although the liver transplantation completely removes the diseased liver, the extrahepatic tissue and blood are inevitably left with a small amount of residual virus, which causes the reinfection of HBV in liver. It was reported that the recurrence rate of hepatitis B after liver transplantation for hepatitis B-related liver disease is up to 70–80% in China [74, 75].

The recurrence of hepatitis B is affected by a variety of factors. The use of immunosuppressive agents, preoperative HBV at high replication levels, and without other viral coinfections will increase the rate of postoperative hepatitis B recurrence. In addition, HBV genotypes can also affect the recurrence of hepatitis B after transplantation [76]. Among them, the gene D has the highest recurrence rate.

The study found that patients with HBV reactivation after liver transplantation have more serious hepatocyte damage and faster fibrosis progression [77]. In the short term, it can rapidly develop into fibrous cholestatic hepatitis, cirrhosis, or acute liver failure, resulting in the death of the recipient. Therefore, prevention and treatment of recurrent hepatitis is particularly important.

The practice guideline on prophylaxis and treatment of hepatitis B for liver transplantation in China recommended that HBV DNA should not be detected as much as possible or the HBV DNA level should be minimized before transplantation [78]. Therefore, antiviral drugs such as high-resistance gene barrier NAs (ETV or TDF) should be routinely applied before transplantation. In the liver transplantation, the fully use of HBIG to neutralize HBsAg is a key measure to prevent HBV infected the new liver. After transplantation, the "NAs combined with low-dose HBIG" regimen should be used, which could significantly reduce the risk of hepatitis B recurrence.

HBsAg, HBV DNA, and anti-HBs titers should be frequently detected within 6 months after HBV-related liver transplantation to monitor HBV replication and reinfection, and to determine the dose and frequency of HBIG use. During follow-up, the recipient's anti-HBV titer, which suddenly decreased or wore off, often indicates the recurrence of HBV, so that the therapeutic regimen should be adjusted.

6.2.3 Treatment of HBV reinfection/emerging infection after liver transplantation

HBV reinfection/emerging infection after liver transplantation progresses relatively rapidly, which can lead to liver failure and even death of patients. It is necessary to carry out targeted evaluation and treatment as soon as possible, aiming to rapidly inhibit HBV replication in the short term and to avoid serious liver injury. After the HBV reinfection/emerging infection, HBIG should be discontinued and treated with high-resistance gene barrier NAs, and HBV-resistant mutant genes and regulatory drugs should be tested. Intensive monitoring of HBV DNA levels and liver injury indicators should be performed. When the liver injury indicators are abnormal, the pathological examination of the liver tissue should be considered, and the degree of liver injury and disease progression comprehensively determines whether the liver transplantation should be evaluated again.

In the selection of NAs drugs, in addition to the resistance mutation factors, some scholars believe that HBV genotype should also be a reference factor. According to the difference of HBV gene sequence, it can be divided into 10 genotypes of A-J [79]. In China, HBV infection is mainly B/C type [70]. Numerous studies have shown that the antiviral efficacy of NAs is affected by the HBV genotype. Among them, Chinese literature reports that the antiviral efficacy of NAs is significantly different between HBV gene type B and type C [80–83]. It is summarized in the following table.

At present, the mechanism by which different genotypes of HBV react differently to antiviral drugs is still unclear. Moreover, some scholars have found that the genotype does not affect the antiviral efficacy of the drug, and may be related to the different genotype detection methods used by different researchers and the sample size. In conclusion, there is no consensus on the effect of HBV genotype on the antiviral efficacy of NAs. The specific mechanism and its correlation require further clinical observation and basic experimental research to guide clinical antiviral drug treatment and efficacy judgment (**Table 2**).

6.3 Liver transplantation for alcoholic liver disease

Alcoholic liver disease is caused by long-term heavy drinking. In the early stage, it usually manifests as fatty liver, which in turn can develop into alcoholic hepatitis,

NA species	The difference of the curative effect
ETV/entecavir	B > C
LAM/lamivudine	B > C
ADV/adefovir dipivoxil	No significant difference
TDF/tenofovir disoproxil fumarate	No significant difference
LdT/telbivudine	B > C

Table 2.
NAs make a different curative effect in different HBV genotypes.

liver fibrosis, and cirrhosis. In severe alcohol abuse, extensive hepatocyte necrosis can be induced and even cause liver failure.

According to the 2014 World Health Organization report, the per capita alcohol consumption of Chinese people over the age of 15 is about 6.7 L/year, and 4.8% of the population has alcohol use disorders, including 9.1 and 0.2% for men and women, respectively. Overall, the proportion of Chinese drinkers and the prevalence of alcohol-related liver diseases are on the rise. According to epidemiological survey data of alcohol related liver disease in some provinces, the prevalence of alcohol-related liver disease is 0.50–8.55% [84–86]. From 2000 to 2004, the proportion of alcohol-related liver disease in hospitalized patients with liver disease had increased from 2.4 to 4.3% [87]. The proportion of patients with alcoholic cirrhosis in all patients with cirrhosis increased from 10.8% in 1999 to 24.0% in 2003 [88, 89]. Alcohol-related liver disease has become one of the most important chronic liver disease in China [90].

6.3.1 Indications

It is generally believed that liver transplantation should be considered when patients with alcoholic liver disease meet the following conditions:

(a) Fail to respond to medications.

(b) Liver lesions are severe or end-stage liver disease manifests.

(c) Suspected small liver cancer is present (single nodule <5 cm, 1–3 nodules <3 cm).

(d) No serious alcohol damage in other organs.

(e) After comprehensive factor evaluation, it is determined that there is a lower postoperative recovery of alcohol abuse.

6.3.2 Assess the risk of relapse after transplantation

Studies have shown that the 3-year survival rate of alcoholic patients after liver transplantation is significantly lower than that of nonalcoholic groups [91]. Therefore, in patients with alcoholic liver disease, whether or not successful alcohol withdrawal after liver transplantation becomes the key. Predictors of longer postoperative alcohol withdrawal include: (1) the patient recognizes the severity of alcoholism. (2) The patient has a stable residence. (3) The patient has a stable occupation. (4) The patient has at least one closely related patient to provide spiritual support.

The following factors represent a higher risk of restocking. (1) The patient has had psychological or mental disorders. (2) The patient has unstable personality characteristics. (3) The patient has repeatedly failed to stop drinking. (4) The patient has the habit of drug abuse. (5) The patient's social relationship is isolated. In practice, effective preventive education measures can significantly reduce the patient's redrinking after surgery. At present, the Chinese guidelines are feasible for liver transplantation in patients with alcoholic liver disease who require alcohol withdrawal for 3–6 months before liver transplantation and no serious alcohol damage in liver.

6.4 Liver transplantation for metabolic diseases

Liver is an important metabolic organ of the human body. Therefore, congenital metabolic diseases caused by defects in certain key metabolic steps are often associated with the liver damage. Some genetic metabolic diseases are manifested in liver disease in infants or children. As the disease progresses, nerves, kidneys, heart, bones, vision, hearing, and skin mucosa are damaged. Liver diseases can also aggravated, leading to cirrhosis and liver failure. These diseases are collectively referred to as hereditary metabolic liver disease.

There are many kinds of genetic metabolic diseases, and the etiology is complicated, 50–60% in childhood. At present, there are more than 600 kinds of hereditary metabolic liver diseases, including carbohydrate metabolism disease, amino acid metabolism disease, fatty acid metabolism disease, organic acid metabolism disease, mitochondrial liver disease, lysosomal disease, peroxisome disease, and metal. There are nine categories of metabolic disorders and 1-antitrypsin deficiency.

Liver disease progresses to advanced cirrhosis or liver failure and requires liver transplantation. According to CLTR, 0.69% of the liver transplantation from DCD is caused by hereditary metabolic liver diseases. In living donor liver transplantation, the rate is 4.13%.

The clinical manifestations of genetic metabolic diseases are diverse, and the symptoms are often not limited to the liver. Since some hereditary metabolic liver diseases often involve multiple organ systems, liver transplantation cannot solve the lesions outside the liver, leading to a poor prognosis. There are certain limitations in liver transplantation in this respect. For example, the effect of simple liver transplantation on patients with progressive familial intrahepatic cholestasis type 1 is not ideal. For these diseases, it is often necessary to cooperate with other treatments. For example, for hyperglycinemia, liver transplantation can only improve the clinical symptoms, and patients can continue to excrete succinylacetone in the urine after surgery. Therefore, some cases need to be combined with liver and kidney transplantation to correct metabolic abnormalities.

7. Immunosuppressants for liver transplantation

With the rapid development of liver transplantation technology, immunosuppressive drugs and drug regimens have emerged in endlessly, playing an increasingly important role. Looking back, medical pioneers had to use crude technical means such as whole-body x irradiation. Until the advent of cyclosporine, liver transplantation has gradually become the main stream of treatment for liver failure. Today, drugs like azathioprine have almost withdrawn from the stage of history. More and more novel immunosuppressants and different strategies are coming into view. Understanding each agent's potency and deficiencies is an essential part of clinical practice. No immunosuppressant is universally applicable yet. Patients with renal impairment, malignancy, or autoimmune diseases may need specific agent or regimen. Therefore, individualized treatment is essential. Here, some commonly used immunosuppressants will be briefly introduced and discussed. Emphasis will be placed on the clinical application, rather than the mechanism of agents (**Table 3** and **Figure 5**).

7.1 Calcineurin inhibitors

Cyclosporine and tacrolimus are two well-known calcineurin inhibitors (CNIs). Both of them are discovered from the soil fungus and are mechanistically similar. They can suppress the immune system by inhibiting interleukin 2 (IL2) gene transcription. Cyclosporine's effect is mediated by cyclosporine's association with cyclophilin, while the tacrolimus's effect is mediated by a specific interaction with FK-binding protein-12 (FKBP12), both of which can result in inhibition of the calcium/calmodulin-dependent phosphatase complex calcineurin, hence the designation "calcineurin inhibitor" (or CNI). An important distinction is that the immunosuppressive potency of tacrolimus is estimated to be 100-fold greater on a molar level. Due to their powerful capacity in reducing acute rejection, the CNIs have been playing an important role in immunosuppression regimens postliver transplantation. As it should be noted that most recent trials use tacrolimus monotherapy or tacrolimus-based therapy as the control group, suggesting that tacrolimus is considered the standard against, which other immunosuppressants are compared.

Despite the potency of CNIs, some serious problems remain. The CNIs may have close relationship with renal toxicity, HCV reinfection, hepatocellular carcinoma recurrence, and some other negative effects [92–94]. So how to use CNIs properly in liver transplantation is a conundrum. At present, to perform therapeutic drug monitoring to reduce the chance of overdosing is necessary, but not enough. The only reasonable step when facing those complicated cases is to minimize or eliminate CNI use.

7.2 Antimetabolites

As for antimetabolites, what is popular now is mycophenolate mofetil (MMF; Hoffmann La Roche, Basel, Switzerland), which is a prodrug of mycophenolic acid (MPA). It takes effect through inhibiting inosine-59-monophosphate dehydrogenase (IMPDH), an important enzyme for de novo synthesis of guanosine nucleotides. Thanks to Sollinger, MMF was brought to the clinic in the early 1990s and used as an immunosuppressant from then on.

Another prodrug of MPA being used clinically is referred to as enteric-coated mycophenolate sodium (ECMPS; Novartis, Basel, Switzerland). Different from MMF, EC-MPS is not rapidly absorbed in the stomach; it is a delayed-release drug formulation that allows release of MPA in the small intestine via a pH-dependent dissolution. The research and development of EC-MPS was trying to solve the well-known gastrointestinal side effects of MMF. However, things are not as smooth as imagined. Studies have not demonstrated fewer side effects with EC-MPS [95].

Due to the renal toxicity of CNI, MMF and EC-MPS are playing an increasing potential role in liver transplantation as they basically have no nephrotoxicity. Several studies have now shown that MMF and EC-MPS are superior to CNIs in terms of renal function, at the cost of a higher rejection rate [96]. For now, compromise is inevitable in such situation. Regimens like "MMF/EC-MPS +low dose CNIs" are acceptable [97].

As mentioned above, MMF and EC-MPS are not without side effects. Both gastrointestinal disorders and hematological suppression are concerns that cannot be ignored.

By the way, azathioprine (AZA) is another antimetabolite that has left an important part in the history of liver transplantation. Though its role for preventing rejection has been almost completely replaced by MMF/EC-MPS, some researches demonstrated that AZA may have some kind of anti-HCV effects [98, 99].

Immunosuppressants		**Action**	**Merits**	**Demerits**
T cell activation inhibitors	Cyclosporine	Inhibits calcineurin via cyclophilin, blocking IL2 transcription	• Reliable antirejection effect • Rich experience in using	• Renal toxicity • Malignancy • Diabetes, fibrosis...
	Tacrolimus	Inhibits calcineurin via FKBP12, blocking IL2 transcription		
T cell proliferation inhibitors	MPA prodrugs	IMPDH inhibitor: enzyme required for de novo synthesis of guanosine nucleotides, required for lymphocyte proliferation	• Low renal toxicity	• Acute rejection • Gastrointestinal side effects
	mTOR inhibitors	mTOR blockade prevents IL2-induced T cell proliferation	• Less renal toxicity	• Wound healing↓, mouth ulcers, hyperlipidemia
	Azathioprine	Inhibits purine synthesis, thereby blocking immune cell proliferation	• Cheap • Possible anti-HCV effects	• Relative weak immunosuppression

Note: AZA: azathioprine.

Table 3.
Comparison of common immunosuppressive agents.

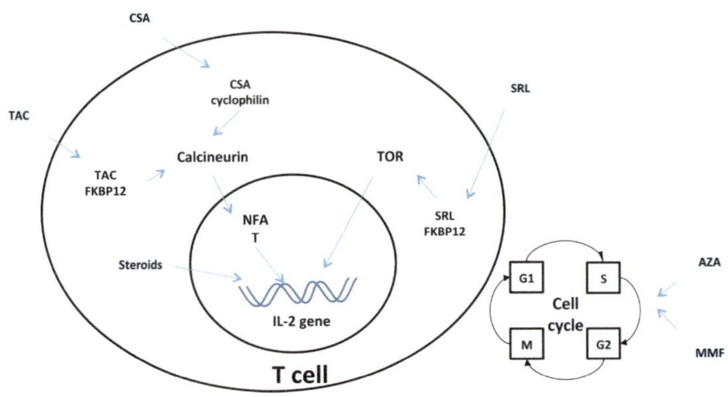

Figure 5.
The mechanism of common immunosuppressive agents.

7.3 mTOR inhibitors

Mammalian target of rapamycin (mTOR) inhibitors include sirolimus (rapamycin; Wyeth) and everolimus (a rapamycin derivative; Novartis). Rapamycin was first discovered in soil from Easter Island (Rapa Nui). Researchers were trying to find its fungi inhibiting ability while accidentally found its immunosuppressive effect. Rapamycin can bind to FKBP12 and form FKBP12 immunosuppressive complex, which can bind to and inhibit the activity of mTOR, thus inhibiting the development of G1 to S phase in cell cycle. Unlike the CNI effects, rapamycin allows T cell activation, but prevents cells from proliferating in response to IL2.

mTOR inhibitors have been approved for use in renal and heart transplantation in combination with CNIs, but not in liver transplantation so far. The use of mTOR inhibitors may cause several adverse reactions:

(a) It may be related to the development of early posttransplant hepatic artery thrombosis, though not confirmed [100, 101].

(b) It may elevate blood lipids (cholesterol).

(c) It may cause wound-healing delays, leg edema and mouth ulcers.

(d) However, this is not to say that mTOR inhibitors have no advantage in liver transplantation.

(e) It may reduce early renal dysfunction compared to CNIs.

(f) It may promote liver allograft tolerance compared to CNIs [102, 103].

(g) It has antitumor effects compared to CNIs [104, 105].

(h) It may have antifibrosis effect [106].

All in all, although mTOR inhibitors are not approved for use in liver transplantation yet, they have good reasons for further investigation.

7.4 Steroids

No doubt, steroids have made great contributions through the development of liver transplantation. For many years, they have been fighting against rejection.

While as always the case, their utilization today is controversial. On one hand, corticosteroids have a wide range of immunosuppressive properties:

(a) Inhibit arachidonic acid metabolism

(b) Affect antigen presentation by dendritic cells

(c) Inhibit IL1-dependent lymphocyte activation by decreasing IL1 transcription

Their broad spectrum of effects provides excellent anti-inflammatory activity that often reverses ongoing allograft rejection.

Of course, their side effects are also well known such as diabetes, hypertension, osteoporosis, obesity, etc. Besides, researches also suggested that high-dose steroids may exacerbate HCV infection and fibrosis, especially when used as pulse therapy for antirejection treatment [107]. Thus, how to use steroids in a proper way is still a pending problem. A variety of steroid-free/minimization immunosuppressive protocols in liver transplantation are under evaluation [108].

7.5 Other promising immunosuppressants or therapy

Due to space limitations, we did not talk about biologic agents like ATG and basiliximab, and will not discuss those promising agents such as belatacept, alemtuzumab and efalizumab, or cellular-based therapy, which may be widely used in liver transplantation in the future. For details, readers can refer to [109].

7.6 Common solutions and suggestions

Tacrolimus-based therapy: "Tac + MMF + steroids" or "Tac + steroids."

Day 0 (the day of the operation): methylprednisolone 500 mg, intravenous, intraoperative; no Tac.

Postoperation: Tac 0.05 mg/(kg*d), twice, later adjust the dose according to blood concentration; methylprednisolone, gradually decrease the dosage, and on day 7 changed to prednisone 20 mg, oral administration; MMF 1.5–2 mg/d, twice.

About 24–48 hours after Tac administration, blood concentration should be tested, and together with other clinical results adjust the Tac dosage.

Steroids withdrawal strategy: day 0, methylprednisolone 500 mg, intravenous, intraoperative; day 1, 240 mg; then decrease 40 mg every day; day 7, change to prednisone 20 mg, oral administration. 1 month postoperation, start to decrease prednisone dosage, decrease 2.5 mg every 2 weeks. For hepatic cancer and hepatitis C recipients, the process of reducing the dosage should be fast. While for the primary biliary cirrhosis and combined liver kidney transplantation recipients, the process should be slower. In addition, gastric protective drugs should be used when steroids are used.

For better-individualized medication, we have to understand the merits and demerits of each immunosuppressant available for liver transplantation, along with each patient's condition. On this individualized basis, our ultimate goal is to minimize or even eliminate long-term pharmacological immunosuppression in liver transplantation recipients. Though difficult, it is worth the effort.

8. Postoperative follow-up of liver transplantation

Nowadays, with the improvement of the surgical techniques of liver transplantation and the update of immunosuppressive agents, liver transplantation in china is getting more and more mature, which has already been in line with the international standards, approximately 95% of patients can safely get through the perioperative period and discharge from hospital [110, 111]. With the increasing of cases of liver transplantation and the prolongation of life span, the patients' long-term treatment and follow-up work have been paid more and more attention by experts and related scholars.

The follow-up of liver transplantation is a long and complex work, which is mainly characterized by large data volume, individual differences, and long follow-up period (generally, lifelong follow-up). An efficient and reasonable follow-up system can not only improve the efficiency of the transplant center, but can also increase the rate of survival of patients. With the gradual standardization of liver transplantation, an ideal postoperative follow-up system has become an important indicator of a mature liver transplantation center.

8.1 Meaning of regular follow-up

Through regular follow-up, the clinicians can dynamically observe the rehabilitation, mental state and medication situation of liver transplant recipients, and give necessary guidance and health education. In the follow-up, the clinicians can detect and deal with the complications after liver transplantation in time, improve the quality of life, prolong the survival period after the operation. Because the incidence of tumor after transplantation is higher than that of the general population, especially liver transplantation of HCC patients may lead to tumor recurrence and metastasis, follow-up regularly can promptly detect the tumor and give appropriate treatment. Moreover, follow-up is the need of medical model transformation, which makes up for the shortage of medical resources, is a tracking service and also an active service. In today's China acute contradiction between doctors and patients, follow-up is a very good way of communication, which can make the relationship between doctors and patients more harmonious and understand each other more. Meanwhile, collection of information of the regular follow-up can accumulate valuable experience for clinical and scientific research [112].

8.2 Development and method of follow-up in China

Liver transplantation centers in China are in different stages of development, and each center should choose a suitable follow-up method according to its outpatient follow-up volume and staffing. With the increase of liver transplantation cases, our center has established the database for recipients' management and follow-up since 2002, which is constantly updated and improved. In the early stage of liver transplantation, many centers in China lack a sound follow-up system, which is passive and sporadic. In 2008, China Liver Transplantation Registry (CLTR) came into use, the first liver transplantation scientific registration system in China, which is an intelligent data collection and management system in line with the characteristics of organ transplantation in China [48]. It sets up a good platform for clinical evidence-based medicine and the scientific research and provides patients with high-quality medical service at the same time. In our center, we set specialized transplant clinic and establish a complete follow-up procedure (**Figure 6**). The patients should follow the standard follow-up program in the absence of complications, including outpatient frequency and inspection items of follow-up (see **Table 4**) [113, 114]. Because exceeding or insufficient immunosuppressive agent has a negative effect on graft function, its concentration must be monitored regularly (see **Table 5**). In addition, there is a big problem in China now that all the candidates and recipients are lack of health education related with organ

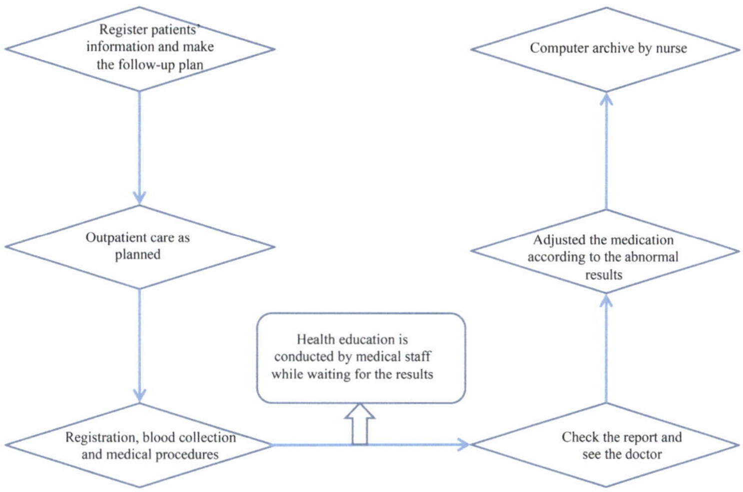

Figure 6.
Follow-up procedure after liver transplantation.

transplantation, which lead to many problems of long survival and better quality of life. Our center is aware of it and gives the patients regular health education during follow-up through PPT, video and handbook, etc. [115, 116].

Inspection items	1–3 m post-LT	3–6 m post-LT	6–12 m post-LT	>12 m post-LT
Blood routine	Once a week	Once 2 weeks	Once a month	Once half year
Liver function	Once a week	Once 2 weeks	Once a month	Once half year
Renal function	Once a week	Once 2 weeks	Once a month	Once half year
Blood glucose and lipids levels	Once a week	Once 2 weeks	Once a month	Once half year
Blood coagulation function	Once a week	Once 2 weeks	Once a month	Once half year
Immunosuppressive agent concentration	Once a week	Once 2 weeks	Once a month	Once half year
HBsAg (for chronic hepatitis B patients)	Once a month		Once half year	
HBV-DNA (for chronic hepatitis B patients)	Once a month		Once half year	
HCV-DNA	Once a month		Once half year	
AFP (for hepatocellular carcinoma patients)	Once a month		Once half year	
Color ultrasound of transplanted liver	Once a month		Once half year	
Chest film or lung CT	Once a month		Once half year	
CT and MRCP	Once 3 months		Once half year	

Abbreviation: m, month; post-LT, post liver transplantation.

Table 4.
Frequency and inspection items of follow-up.

	1 D–1 Mpost-LT	1–3 Mpost-LT	3–12 Mpost-LT	>12 Mpost-LT
Fk506 C_0 (ng/mL)	8–10	6–8	6–8	5–7
CSA C_0 (ng/mL)	200–350	150–300	100–250	>50
CSA C_2 (ng/mL)	1000–1500	800–1200	600–1000	>400
SIR C_0 (ng/mL)	5–8	4–8	4–8	3–6

Abbreviation: C0, the minimal concentration; C2, peak plasma concentration.

Table 5.
Immunosuppressive agents concentration based on postoperative time.

As is well known, the success of liver transplant surgery only means the beginning of a new life for patients. The long-term survival of liver transplant recipients depends not only on the surgical skills of surgeons, but also on the high quality and efficient follow-up after liver transplantation. With the increase in the number of liver transplantation and the application of CLTR, the experts and scholars in China will have more experience to help the patients benefit from liver transplantation.

9. Conclusion and future perspectives

After decades of efforts, the liver transplantation in Mainland China has made many achievements. The number of cases has ranked second in the world, and the quality and survival rate are no different from those of advanced countries; since 2010, China's organ donation work has been gradually carried out, and the source of liver transplant donors has transitioned from relying on judicial channels to DCDs and relative living donors. Before 2015, DCD work has not been widely carried out in the country. For some time, due to the shortage of donors, the proportion of living relatives has increased significantly (**Figures** 7 and **8**), but with the development of DCD work, DCD has become the main source of liver, which better alleviated the problem of organ shortage, meanwhile many shortcoming and problems have been exposed in the DCD era.

(1) The main primary disease of liver transplantation in current China is still HBV-related disease. China is a large HBV country, and patients requiring liver transplantation are increasing year by year. Although DCD donors alleviate the shortage of donors to a certain extent, it is necessary for Chinese health management departments to pay more attention to the prevention and treatment of HBV and related research work. For transplant experts, more work and research is needed on HBV treatment and prevention of recurrence before and after transplantation.

(2) The proportion of liver cancer liver transplants in China is high (**Figures 9** and **10**). How to develop a liver transplantation standard suitable for liver cancer in China, how to reduce the recurrence of liver cancer after transplantation, prolong the survival time, and how to effectively combine with immunosuppressant are also problems faced by Chinese physicians.

(3) Legal regulations are not yet complete. China has not established a brain death law, and the relevant transplant laws and regulations are also quite lacking.

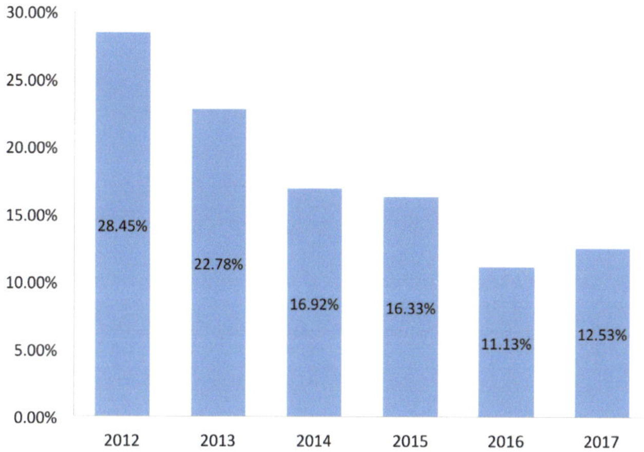

Figure 7.
Proportion of living donor liver transplantation (data from CLTR).

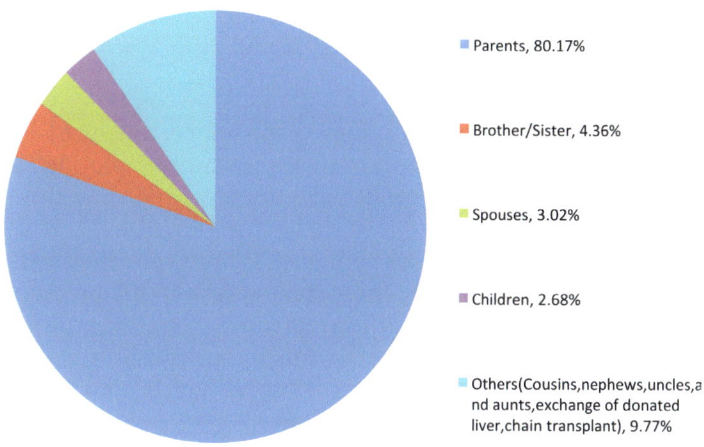

Figure 8.
The categories of living donors (data from CLTR).

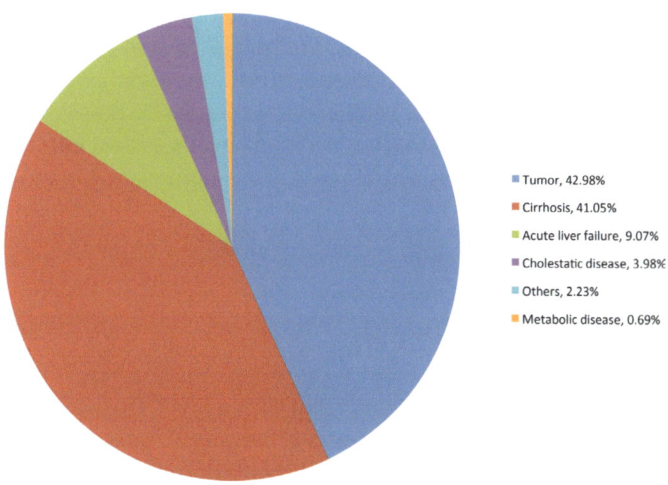

Figure 9.
2010–2017 Primary disease statistics of DCD liver transplant recipients (data from CLTR).

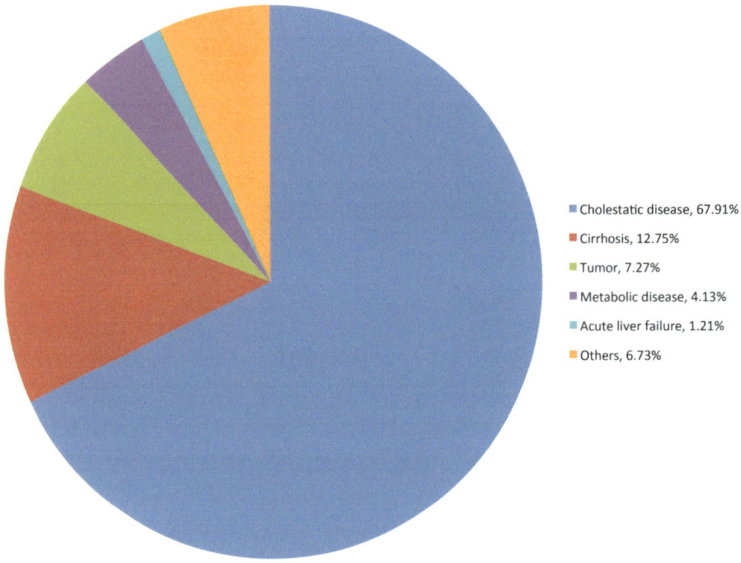

Figure 10.
2010–2017 Primary disease statistics of living donor liver transplant recipients (data from CLTR).

The corresponding management system is still not perfect. The Chinese government and transplant experts are also constantly exploring and working hard on these issues.

(4) DCD-related work needs to be strengthened. China's contribution rate per million populations is very low, only about three cases per million people. In order to better carry out DCD work, it is necessary to increase the positive publicity of organ donation, further improve the donation, acquisition and distribution system, and establish effective services for transplant-related institutions. These are issues that China still needs to solve.

China's liver transplantation is facing enormous challenges and opportunities. It not only faces legal issues, sociology, ethics, and many other issues in donor donation, but also requires surgeons to refine and continuously improve surgical methods. More related researches needed to be done by transplant scholars. The entry criteria for liver transplant recipients and the induction of human immune tolerance in accordance with China's national conditions also depend on further research by domestic transplant workers, and the solution to these problems will be tortuous and difficult. We believe that through the long-term joint efforts of the Chinese transplanting colleagues, China's liver transplantation will have a brighter future.

Acknowledgements

We thank Prof. Zheng Shu-sen from liver transplantation center of the first hospital of Zhejiang University and workers from China Liver Transplantation Register (CLTR) for their technique support and data providing. This work was supported by grants from the National Natural Science Foundation of China (no. 81771722) to YZM and (no. 81700658) to QZ, and the Natural Science Foundation of Hunan Province (no. 2016JJ4105) to QZ.

Conflict of interest

No conflict of interest.

Author details

Yingzi Ming*, Quan Zhuang, Baoren Tu, Gangcheng Kong, Hao Li, Ying Niu, Bo Peng, Junhui Li, Meng Yu and Min Yang
Transplantation Center of the 3rd Xiangya Hospital, Central South University, Engineering and Technology Research Center for Transplantation Medicine of National Ministry of Health, Changsha, Hunan, China

*Address all correspondence to: myz_china@aliyun.com

References

[1] Chen GH. Liver transplantation in Mainland China: Past, present and future. Organ Transplantation. 2010;**1**(1):5-6

[2] Chen H, Zang YJ, Zhu XW, Shen ZY. A brief history of liver transplantation. Chinese Journal of Medical History. 2006;**36**(4):227-230

[3] Notice of the General Office of the Ministry of Health on Doing a Good Job in the Registration of Subjects for Human Organ Transplantation. Issued by General Office of the Ministry of Health. Vol. 87. 2007

[4] Regulations on Organ Transplantation. State Council Order No. 491

[5] Zheng SS, Yu J, Zhang W. Current development of liver transplantation in China. Journal of Clinical hepatology. 2014;**30**(1):2-4

[6] Huo F, Li P. The past, current situation, and future of DCD Liver transplantation. Journal of Hepatobiliary Surgery. 2014;**22**(2):84-86

[7] Organ Donation after Cardiac Death Classification Standard of the Ministry of Health of the People's Republic China. Available from: http://www.moh.gov.cn/publicfiles/business/cmsresources/mohy/fwjgs/cmsrsdocument/doc11852.doc [Accessed: Oct 15, 2011]

[8] Zhu JY, Gao PJ. The current situation of organ donation after citizen death liver transplantation. Chinese Journal of Hepatobiliary Surgery (Electronic Edition). 2016;**5**(5):273-276

[9] Huang JF. The development path and expectation of China organ donation. Medical Journal of Wuhan University. 2016;**37**(4):517-522

[10] Rao W. A Brief Introduction of Liver Transplantation Development Path in China. Available from: www.haodf.com

[11] Guo YH. The number of liver transplantation in China last year. Chinese Family News. June 28, 2018

[12] Wang XH, Li GQ. The current situation and challenges facing by liver transplantation in China. Chinese Journal of Digestive Surgery. 2013;**12**(9):641-643

[13] China Organ Donation Administrative Center. December 31, 2016

[14] Huang JF, Li ZH, Guo ZY, HeXS. The development path of organ donation in China. Chinese Journal of Critical Care and Intensive Care Medicine. 2017;**3**(2):81-84

[15] Fu B, Yi S, Tang H, Yi M, Meng W, Zhang T, et al. Experience of quality evaluation and function maintenance of donor liver from organ donation after citizen's death. Organ Transplantation. 2016;**7**:215-218. DOI: 10.3969/j.issn.1674-7445.2016.03.011

[16] Li D, Xu C, Li Z, Guan G, Zhang B. Multifactor analysis on the quality of DCD donor liver. Practical Journal of Organ Transplantation (Electronic Version). 2018;**6**:25-29. DOI: 10.3969/j.issn.2095-5332.2018.01.007

[17] Shu Z, Xiang P, Zheng S. Quality assessment and protection of liver donated by cardiac death donor. Chinese Journal of Organ Transplantation. 2014;**35**:698-700. DOI: 10.3760/cma.j.issn.0254-1785.2014.11.016

[18] Duan X, Zheng S. Quality assessment of donation after cardiac death liver. Chinese Journal of Transplantation (Electronic Edition). 2015;**9**:38-41. DOI: 10.3877/cma.j.issn.1674-3903.2015.01.009

[19] Xia L. The problems in DCD donor liver preoperative evaluation. Journal of Hepatobiliary Surgery.

2017;**25**:241-243. DOI: 10.3969/j.issn.1006-4761.2017.04.001

[20] Xia W, Ke Q, Wang Y, Feng X, Guo H, Wang W, et al. Donation after cardiac death liver transplantation: Graft quality evaluation based on pretransplant liver biopsy. Liver Transplantation. 2015;**21**:838-846. DOI: 10.1002/lt.24123

[21] Liu Z, Zhao H, Geng X. Progress in rapid pathological examination in liver grafts selection. Chinese Journal of Organ Transplantation. 2014;**35**:760-762. DOI: 10.3760/cma.j.issn.0254-1785.2014.12.014

[22] Shi X, Fu Z, Ding G, Ni Z, Wang Z, Guo W, et al. Rapid evaluation of quality of liver and perfusion at the liver graft harvesting. Journal of Hepatobiliary Surgery. 2005;**13**:184-186. DOI: 10.3969/j.issn.1006-4761.2005.03.009

[23] Zhang Y, Yang Q, Lv H, Fu B, Liu W. Application of metabolomics in the evaluation of liver grafts from cardiac dead donors. Organ Transplantation. 2017;**8**:472-475. DOI: 10.3969/j.issn.1674-7445.2017.06.012

[24] Zheng SS, Ye QF, Li JH, Xu X, Xie HY, Wang YF. Chinese expert consensus on organ protection in transplantation. Chinese Archives of General Surgery (Electronic Edition). 2016;**10**(5):315-323. DOI: 10.3760/cma.j.issn.1007-8118.2016.09.001

[25] Cheng Y. Application of mechanical perfusion in liver transplantation. Organ Transplantation. 2016;7:390-393. DOI: 10.3969/j.issn.1674-7445.2016.05.012

[26] Reich DJ, Mulligan DC, Abt PL, et al. ASTS recommended practice guidelines for controlled donation after cardiac death organ procurement and transplantation. American Journal of Transplantation. 2009;**9**(9):2004-2011

[27] Ye SJ, Ming YZ, Ye QF, et al. Experience of bench preparation of donor liver in liver transplantation. Chinese Journal of General Surgery. 2007;**16**(3):261-264

[28] Starzl TE, Iwatsuki S, Van Thiel DH. Evolution of liver transplantation. Hepatology. 1982;**2**(5):614-636

[29] Özgün G, Haberal Reyhan N, Özdemir BH, Haberal M. Liver transplant for hepatocellular carcinoma: Pathologic point of view. Experimental and Clinical Transplantation. 2017;**15**(Suppl 2):50-54

[30] Zheng SS, Liang TB. Experience in classical orthotopic liver transplantation. Surgical Theory and Practice. 2002;**7**(2):91-93

[31] Yassen AM, Elsarraf WR, Elmorshedi MA. Short-term effects of extracorporeal graft rinse versus circulatory graft rinse in living donor liver transplantation. A prospective randomized controlled trial. Transplant International. 2017;**30**(7):725-733

[32] Zheng SS, Liang TB. Discussion on venous bypass and non-flow problems in orthotopic liver transplantation. Chinese Journal of Basic and Clinical Medicine. 2002;**9**(4):217-218

[33] Zheng SS, Huang DS, Wu J. Classical orthotopic liver transplantation without extracorporeal venous-venous bypass. Chinese Journal of Surgery. 2002;**40**(5):326-328

[34] Xia Q. The surgical essentials of classic orthotopic liver transplantation. Journal of Hepatobiliary Surgery. 2007;**15**(5):326-327

[35] Zheng SS, Bai XL, Liang TB, Yan S, Wang WL, Shen Y, et al. Microsurgical reconstruction of hepatic artery variability in liver transplantation. Chinese Journal of General Surgery. 2004;**19**(1):7-9

[36] Ma Y, He XS, Zhu XF, Wang GD, Wang D, Ping W, et al. Techniques for orthotopic liver transplantation

for biliary reconstruction. Chinese Journal of Practical Surgery. 2008;**28**(3):200-202

[37] Ye QF. The evolution of piggyback liver transplantation and the development status of international piggyback liver transplantation. Chinese Journal of Modern Medicine. 2004;**14**(13):6-9

[38] Nishida S, Nakamura N, Vaidya A, Levi DM, Kato T, Nery JR, et al. Piggyback technique in adult orthotopic liver transplantation: An analysis of 1067 liver transplants at a single center. Hepato Pancreato Biliary. 2006;**8**(3):182-188

[39] Schembri V, Cassinotto C, Panaro F. Challenging TIPS in liver transplant recipients: The pull-through technique to address piggyback anastomosis. Cardiovascular and Interventional Radiology. 2018;**41**(5):804-810

[40] Lauro A, Vaidya A. Role of "reduced-size" liver/bowel grafts in the "abdominal wall transplantation" era. World Journal of Gastrointestinal Surgery. 2017;**9**(9):186-192

[41] Ji HF, Wang WL, Shen Y. Reduced-size liver transplantation for glycogen storage disease. Hepatobiliary & Pancreatic Diseases International. 2009;**8**(1):106-108

[42] Oswari H, Lynch SV, Fawcett J, Strong RW, Ee LC. Outcomes of split versus reduced-size grafts in pediatric liver transplantation. Journal of Gastroenterology and Hepatology. 2005;**20**(12):1850-1854

[43] Zhu ZJ, Zeng ZG. Research progress in assisted liver transplantation. Journal of Clinical Hepatology. 2015;**31**(12):2020-2022

[44] Yang YX, Dou KF. Selection and implementation of assisted liver transplantation. Journal of Hepatobiliary Surgery. 2013;**21**(4):247-250

[45] Kim SH, Hwang S, Ha TY, Song GW, Jung DH, Ahn CS, et al. Usability of cryopreserved aortic allografts for middle hepatic vein reconstruction during living-donor liver transplantation. Journal of Gastrointestinal Surgery. 2016;**20**(5):1049-1055. DOI: 10.1007/s11605-015-3048-0

[46] Figiel W, Grat M, Wronka KM, Patkowski W, Krasnodebski M, Masior L, et al. Reoperations for intraabdominal bleeding following deceased donor liver transplantation. Polski Przeglad Chirurgiczny. 2016;**88**(4):196-201. DOI: 10.1515/pjs-2016-0051

[47] Li C, Wen TF, Yan LN, Li B. Risk factors for abdominal bleeding after living-donor liver transplant. Experimental and Clinical Transplantation. 2014;**12**(5):424-428. DOI: 10.6002/ect.2013.0223

[48] Wei Q, Gao F, Zhuang R, Ling Q, Ke Q, Wu J, et al. A national report from China liver transplant registry: Steroid avoidance after liver transplantation for hepatocellular carcinoma. Chinese Journal of Cancer Research. 2017;**29**(5):426-437. DOI: 10.21147/j.issn.1000-9604.2017.05.07

[49] Lui SK, Garcia CR, Mei X, Gedaly R. Re-transplantation for hepatic artery thrombosis: A national perspective. World Journal of Surgery. 2018;**42**(10):3357-3363. DOI: 10.1007/s00268-018-4609-7

[50] Mourad MM, Liossis C, Gunson BK, Mergental H, Isaac J, Muiesan P, et al. Etiology and management of hepatic artery thrombosis after adult liver transplantation. Liver Transplantation. 2014;**20**(6):713-723. DOI: 10.1002/lt.23874

[51] Pulitano C, Joseph D, Sandroussi C, Verran D, Strasser SI, Shackel NA, et al. Hepatic artery stenosis after liver transplantation: Is endovascular

treatment always necessary? Liver Transplantation. 2015;**21**(2):162-168. DOI: 10.1002/lt.24043

[52] Ma L, Lu Q, Luo Y. Vascular complications after adult living donor liver transplantation: Evaluation with ultrasonography. World Journal of Gastroenterology. 2016;**22**(4):1617-1626. DOI: 10.3748/wjg.v22.i4.1617

[53] Boleslawski E, Bouras AF, Truant S, Liddo G, Herrero A, Badic B, et al. Hepatic artery ligation for arterial rupture following liver transplantation: A reasonable option. American Journal of Transplantation. 2013;**13**(4):1055-1062. DOI: 10.1111/ajt.12135

[54] Senter-Zapata M, Khan AS, Subramanian T, Vachharajani N, Dageforde LA, Wellen JR, et al. Patient and graft survival: Biliary complications after liver transplantation. Journal of the American College of Surgeons. 2018;**226**(4):484-494. DOI: 10.1016/j.jamcollsurg.2017.12.039

[55] Coelho JCU, Leite LO, Molena A, Freitas ACT, Matias JEF. Biliary complications after liver transplantation. Arquivos Brasileiros de Cirurgia Digestiva. 2017;**30**(2):127-131. DOI: 10.1590/0102-6720201700020011

[56] Ye S, Dong JH, Duan WD, Ji WB, Liang YR. The preliminary study on procurement biliary convergence from donors with complicated bile duct variant in emergency right lobe living donor liver transplantation. Journal of Clinical and Experimental Hepatology. 2017;**7**(1):33-41. DOI: 10.1016/j.jceh.2016.09.016

[57] Li DW, Lu TF, Hua XW, Dai HJ, Cui XL, Zhang JJ, et al. Risk factors for new onset diabetes mellitus after liver transplantation: A meta-analysis. World Journal of Gastroenterology. 2015;**21**(20):6329-6340. DOI: 10.3748/wjg.v21.i20.6329

[58] Watt KD, Charlton MR. Metabolic syndrome and liver transplantation: A review and guide to management. Journal of Hepatology. 2010;**53**(1):199-206. DOI: 10.1016/j.jhep.2010.01.040

[59] Zheng J, Wang WL. Risk factors of metabolic syndrome after liver transplantation. Hepatobiliary & Pancreatic Diseases International. 2015;**14**(6):582-587

[60] Longenecker JC, Waheed S, Bandak G, Murakami CA, McMahon BA, Gelber AC, et al. Hyperuricemia after orthotopic liver transplantation: Divergent associations with progression of renal disease, incident end-stage renal disease, and mortality. BMC Nephrology. 2017;**18**(1):103. DOI: 10.1186/s12882-017-0518-5

[61] Neal DA, Tom BD, Gimson AE, Gibbs P, Alexander GJ. Hyperuricemia, gout, and renal function after liver transplantation. Transplantation. 2001;**72**(10):1689-1691

[62] Transplantation Chinese Society of Organ, Section of Organ Transplantation Chinese Society of Surgery, Doctors Chinese College of Transplant. The Chinese clinical practice guideline on liver transplantation for hepatocellular carcinoma (2014 edition). Practical Journal of Organ Transplantation (Electronic Version). 2015;**3**:66-71

[63] Zheng SS, Xu X, Wu J, Chen J, Wang WL, Zhang M, et al. Liver transplantation for hepatocellular carcinoma: Hangzhou experiences. Transplantation. 2008;**85**(12):1726-1732. DOI: 10.1097/TP.0b013e31816b67e4

[64] Fan J, Zhou J, Xu Y, Qiu SJ, Wu ZQ, Yu Y, et al. Indication of liver transplantation for hepatocellular carcinoma: Shanghai Fudan criteria. Zhonghua Yi Xue Za Zhi. 2006;**86**(18):1227-1231

[65] Clavien PA, Lesurtel M, Bossuyt PM, Gores GJ, Langer B, Perrier A, et al. Recommendations for liver transplantation for hepatocellular carcinoma: An international consensus conference report. The Lancet Oncology. 2012;**13**(1):e11-e22. DOI: 10.1016/S1470-2045(11)70175-9

[66] European Association for the Study of the Liver, European Organisation for Research, Treatment of Cancer. EASL-EORTC clinical practice guidelines: Management of hepatocellular carcinoma. Journal of Hepatology. 2012;**56**(4):908-943. DOI: 10.1016/j.jhep.2011.12.001

[67] Mazzaferro V, Llovet JM, Miceli R, Bhoori S, Schiavo M, Mariani L, et al. Predicting survival after liver transplantation in patients with hepatocellular carcinoma beyond the Milan criteria: A retrospective, exploratory analysis. The Lancet Oncology. 2009;**10**(1):35-43. DOI: 10.1016/S1470-2045(08)70284-5

[68] Zimmerman MA, Ghobrial RM, Tong MJ, Hiatt JR, Cameron AM, Hong J, et al. Recurrence of hepatocellular carcinoma following liver transplantation: A review of preoperative and postoperative prognostic indicators. Archives of Surgery. 2008;**143**(2):182-188; discussion 8. DOI: 10.1001/archsurg.2007.39

[69] Liang X, Bi S, Yang W, Wang L, Cui G, Cui F, et al. Evaluation of the impact of hepatitis B vaccination among children born during 1992-2005 in China. The Journal of Infectious Diseases. 2009;**200**(1):39-47. DOI: 10.1086/599332

[70] Liang X, Bi S, Yang W, Wang L, Cui G, Cui F, et al. Epidemiological serosurvey of hepatitis B in China--declining HBV prevalence due to hepatitis B vaccination. Vaccine. 2009;**27**(47):6550-6557. DOI: 10.1016/j.vaccine.2009.08.048

[71] Yuan-Sheng C, Li LI, Fu-Qiang CUI, Wen-Ge X, Lu W, Zhi-Yuan JIA, et al. A sero-epidemiological study on hepatitis C in China. Chinese Journal of Epidemiology. 2011;**9**:888-891. DOI: 10.3760/cma.j.issn.0254-6450.2011.09.009

[72] Chinese Society of Hepatology, Chinese Medical Asso., Chinese Society of Infectious Diseases, Chinese Med. The guideline of prevention and treatment for chronic hepatitis B: A 2015 update. Journal of Clinical Hepatology. 2015;**12**:1941-1960. DOI: 10.3969/j.issn.1001-5256.2015.12.002

[73] Hepatology Chinese Society of Diseases Chinese Society of Infectious. The guideline of prevention and treatment for hepatitis C: A 2015 update. Chinese Hepatology. 2015;**49**(12):933-1006. DOI: 10.3969/j.issn.1008-1704.2015.12.002

[74] Yuan G, Wentao W, Ziqiang L, Gendong T, Lei R, Kai S, et al. Hepatitis B vaccination: A new strategy to prevent hepatitis B recurrence after liver transplantation for hepatitis B virus-related recipients. Chinese Journal of Hepatobiliary Surgery. 2015;**10**:668-670. DOI: 10.3760/cma.j.issn.1007-8118.2015.10.006

[75] Liu G, Chen G, Sun J, Tang G, Wang W, Zhu S. Analysis of lamivudine combined with low-dose hepatitis B immunoglobulin for prevention and treatment of hepatitis B recurrence after liver transplantation. China Practical Medical. 2014;**36**:117-118

[76] Jurim O, Martin P, Shaked A, Goldstein L, Millis JM, Calquhoun SD, et al. Liver transplantation for chronic hepatitis B in Asians. Transplantation. 1994;**57**(9):1393-1395

[77] Yin-Jie GAO, Han-Wei LI, Jing-Min Z, Min Z, Bo JIN, Fan-Ping M. Clinicopathological analysis of HBV recurrence in post-liver transplantation patients. Chinese

Journal of Organ Transplantation. 2011;**8**:477-480. DOI: 10.3760/cma.j.issn.0254-1785.2011.08.008

[78] Chinese Society of Organ Transplantation, Chinese, Chinese Society of Hepatology, Chinese Medical Ass. The practice guideline on prophylaxis and treatment of hepatitis B for liver transplantation in China (2016 edition). Journal of Clinical Hepatology. 2017;**2**:213-220. DOI: 10.3969/j.issn.1001-5256.2017.02.002

[79] Liu CJ, Kao JH. Global perspective on the natural history of chronic hepatitis B: Role of hepatitis B virus genotypes A to J. Seminars in Liver Disease. 2013;**33**(2):97-102. DOI: 10.1055/s-0033-1345716

[80] Xian Y, Cheng S. Progress in research and application of hepatitis B virus genotyping. International Journal of Virology. 2016;**4**:285-288. DOI: 10.3760/cma.j.issn.1673-4092.2016.04.021

[81] Yang L, Peng X, Zhao Y, Zhao P, Ma Y, Yang F. Relationship of HBV genotypes to changes of liver biopsies and to responses to antiviral therapy of nucleoside analogs. Journal of Clinical Hepatology. 2012;**2**:120-122. DOI: 10.3969/j.issn.1672-5069.2012.02.013

[82] Lu D, Zhao L. Relationship between hepatitis B virus genotype and antiviral drug efficacy. Medical Journal of West China. 2005;**4**:389-391. DOI: 10.3969/j.issn.1672-3511.2005.04.064

[83] Lin T, Chen L, Kong J. Different effects of tenofovir treatment with different HBV genotypes in HBeAg positive chronic hepatitis B. China Foreign Medical Treatment. 2017;**23**:38-40. DOI: 10.16662/j.cnki.1674-0742.2017.23.038

[84] Wang H, Ma L, Yin Q, Zhang X, Zhang C. Prevalence of alcoholic liver disease and its association with socioeconomic status in North-Eastern China. Alcoholism, Clinical and Experimental Research. 2014;**38**(4):1035-1041. DOI: 10.1111/acer.12321

[85] Huang S, Dai S, Zhang X, Yu Y, Tan M, Yi C. Survey of epidemiological investigation of alcoholic liver disease in Hunan Province. Journal of Chinese Physician. 2005;**3**:426-427. DOI: 10.3760/cma.j.issn.1008-1372.2005.03.080

[86] Zhou YJ, Li YY, Nie YQ, Ma JX, Lu LG, Shi SL, et al. Prevalence of fatty liver disease and its risk factors in the population of South China. World Journal of Gastroenterology. 2007;**13**(47):6419-6424

[87] Group Chinese Alcoholic Liver Disease Investigation Collaboration. Management of malignant biliary hilar obstruction with multiple stents. Chinese Journal of Digestion. 2007;**4**:231-234. DOI: 10.3760/j.issn:0254-1432.2007.04.005

[88] Liu Y, Chi B. Clinical analysis on 237 cases with alcoholic liver cirrhosis. Jilin Medical Journal. 2004;**2**:40-42. DOI: 10.3969/j.issn.1004-0412.2004.02.016

[89] Wang H, Wang J. Study on the association of hepatitis virus infection and alcoholic liver cirrhosis (a clinic study on 182 patients with alcoholic liver disease). Journal of Norman Bethune University of Medical Science. 1998;**6**:652-653

[90] Wang FS, Fan JG, Zhang Z, Gao B, Wang HY. The global burden of liver disease: The major impact of China. Hepatology (Baltimore, MD). 2014;**60**(6):2099-2108. DOI: 10.1002/hep.27406

[91] Pfitzmann R, Schwenzer J, Rayes N, Seehofer D, Neuhaus R, Nussler NC. Long-term survival and predictors of relapse after orthotopic

liver transplantation for alcoholic liver disease. Liver Transplantation. 2007;**13**(2):197-205. DOI: 10.1002/lt.20934

[92] Firpi RJ, Zhu H, Morelli G, et al. Cyclosporine suppresses hepatitis C virus in vitro and increases the chance of a sustained virological response after liver transplantation. Liver Transplantation. 2006;**12**:51-57. DOI: 10.1002/lt.20532

[93] Guba M, von BP, Steinbauer M, et al. Rapamycin inhibits primary and metastatic tumor growth by antiangiogenesis: Involvement of vascular endothelial growth factor. Nature Medicine. 2002;**8**:128-135. DOI: 10.1038/nm0202-128

[94] Koehl GE, Andrassy J, Guba M, et al. Rapamycin protects allografts from rejection while simultaneously attacking tumors in immunosuppressed mice. Transplantation. 2004;**77**:1319-1326

[95] Schmidt H, Brockmann J. MMF to EC-MPS conversion: What makes the difference. Liver Transplantation. 2007;**13**:773-774; author reply 775. DOI: 10.1002/lt.21101

[96] Schlitt HJ, Barkmann A, Böker KH, et al. Replacement of calcineurin inhibitors with mycophenolate mofetil in liver-transplant patients with renal dysfunction: A randomised controlled study. Lancet. 2001;**357**:587-591

[97] Fisher RA, Ham JM, Marcos A, et al. A prospective randomized trial of mycophenolate mofetil with neoral or tacrolimus after orthotopic liver transplantation. Transplantation. 1998;**66**:1616-1621

[98] Stangl JR, Carroll KL, Illichmann M, Striker R. Effect of antimetabolite immunosuppressants on flaviviridae, including hepatitis C virus. Transplantation. 2004;**77**:562-567

[99] Nebbia G, Mattes FM, Sabin CA, et al. Differential effects of prednisolone and azathioprine on the development of human cytomegalovirus replication post liver transplantation. Transplantation. 2007;**84**:605610. DOI: 10.1097/01.tp.0000280555.08651.11

[100] Kneteman NM, Oberholzer J, Al SM, et al. Sirolimus-based immunosuppression for liver transplantation in the presence of extended criteria for hepatocellular carcinoma. Liver Transplantation. 2004;**10**:1301-1311. DOI: 10.1002/lt.20237

[101] Dunkelberg JC, Trotter JF, Wachs M, et al. Sirolimus as primary immunosuppression in liver transplantation is not associated with hepatic artery or wound complications. Liver Transplantation. 2003;**9**:463-468. DOI: 10.1053/jlts.2003.50079

[102] Li Y, Zheng XX, Li XC, Zand MS, Strom TB. Combined costimulation blockade plus rapamycin but not cyclosporine produces permanent engraftment. Transplantation. 1998;**66**:1387-1388

[103] Li Y, Li XC, Zheng XX, Wells AD, Turka LA, Strom TB. Blocking both signal 1 and signal 2 of T-cell activation prevents apoptosis of alloreactive T cells and induction of peripheral allograft tolerance. Nature Medicine. 1999;**5**:1298-1302. DOI: 10.1038/15256

[104] Luan FL, Hojo M, Maluccio M, Yamaji K, Suthanthiran M. Rapamycin blocks tumor progression: Unlinking immunosuppression from antitumor efficacy. Transplantation. 2002;**73**:1565-1572

[105] Guertin DA, Sabatini DM. Defining the role of mTOR in cancer. Cancer Cell. 2007;**12**:9-22. DOI: 10.1016/j.ccr.2007.05.008

[106] Neef M, Ledermann M, Saegesser H, Schneider V, Reichen J. Low-dose oral rapamycin treatment reduces fibrogenesis, improves liver function, and prolongs survival in rats with established liver cirrhosis. Journal of Hepatology. 2006;**45**:786-796. DOI: 10.1016/j.jhep.2006.07.030

[107] Henry SD, Metselaar HJ, Van Dijck J, Tilanus HW. Van Der Laan LJ.Impact of steroids on hepatitis C virus replication in vivo and in vitro. Annals of the New York Academy of Sciences. 2007;**1110**:439-447. DOI: 10.1196/annals.1423.046

[108] Segev DL, Sozio SM, Shin EJ, et al. Steroid avoidance in liver transplantation: Meta-analysis and meta-regression of randomized trials. Liver Transplantation. 2008;**14**:512-525. DOI: 10.1002/lt.21396

[109] Geissler EK, Schlitt HJ. Immunosuppression for liver transplantation. Gut. 2009;**58**:452-463. DOI: 10.1136/gut.2008.163527

[110] Peng S. Improving the level of liver transplantation in China. Zhonghua Yi Xue Za Zhi. 2001;**81**:1089-1090

[111] Huang J, He X, Chen G, Zhu X, Lu M, Wang G, et al. Liver transplantation at the Sun Yat-Sen University of Medical Sciences in China. Chinese Medical Journal. 2002;**115**:543-548

[112] Wang GS, Yang Y, Li H, Jiang N, Fu BS, Jin H, et al. Health-related quality of life after liver transplantation: The experience from a single Chinese center. Hepatobiliary & Pancreatic Diseases International. 2012;**11**:262-266

[113] Xie M, Rao W, Yang T, Deng Y, Zheng H, Pan C, et al. Occult hepatitis B virus infection predicts de novo hepatitis B infection in patients with alcoholic cirrhosis after liver transplantation. Liver International. 2015;**35**:897-904

[114] Jiang W, Li J, Guo Q, Sun J, Chen C, Shen Z. Liver transplantation for hepatocellular carcinoma. Drug Discoveries & Therapeutics. 2015;**9**:331-334

[115] Zheng H, Zhang HM, Zheng WP. Insight and judgment on recurrence of hepatocellular carcinoma after liver transplantation. Zhonghua Gan Zang Bing Za Zhi. 2018;**26**:88-92

[116] Wei L, Chen D, Zhang B, Zhao Y, Liu B, Shi H, et al. Long-term outcome and recurrence of hepatitis B virus following liver transplantation from hepatitis B surface antigen-positive donors in a Chinese population. Journal of Viral Hepatitis. 2018;**00**:1-6

Section 4

How Diagnosis Affects the Type of Hepatic Surgery

Chapter 7

Colorectal Liver Metastases

Julio Wiederkehr, Barbara Wiederkehr
and Henrique Wiederkehr

Abstract

The adenocarcinoma of the colon and rectum (CRC) affects more than 1.3 million patients each year, being the third most common malignancy in the world. Approximately, 30–50% of these patients will present with liver metastasis at the time of diagnosis or will develop metastasis later. The incidence of metastatic CRC (mCRC) is approximately 4.3% at 1 year, 8.7% at 2 years, 12% at 3 years, and 16.5% at 5 years after resection. Recently, the clinical outcome for patients with mCRC has improved, with a median overall survival (OS) for patients with mCRC is approximately 30 months, more than twice of that observed 20 years ago. The treatment approach for patients with colorectal liver metastases should be focused toward complete resection whenever possible, with both oncological and technical criteria being considered. Considering the fact that nearly 80% of patients with mCRC are not candidates for resection at diagnosis, initial treatment options include chemotherapy and locoregional therapies. Associating liver partition and portal vein ligation for staged hepatectomy (ALPPS) has emerged as modification on classic two-staged hepatectomy (TSH) with portal vein embolization. In experienced hepatobiliary centers and in well-selected patients, ALPPS can be performed with low morbidity and minimal mortality, resulting in good intermediate-term survival and excellent quality of life. Multidisciplinary tumor boards should critically scrutinize the best treatment options.

Keywords: colorectal cancer, liver, liver cancer, liver metastasis

1. Introduction

The adenocarcinoma of the colon and rectum (CRC) affect more than 1.3 million patients each year, being the third most common malignancy in the world [1]. Approximately, 30–50% of these patients will present with liver metastasis at the time of diagnosis or will develop metastasis later [2, 3].

Due to the fact that venous drainage of the intestinal tract is via the portal system, the first site of hematogenous spreading is usually the liver. The most common site of metastatic CRC is the liver, occurring in 80% of cases, representing nearly half of all patients with CRC. It is also the single site of metastasis in 20–50% of the cases [2]. The majority of metastatic CRC liver disease will be potentially resectable at the time of diagnosis, approximately 75–80% of cases [3]. Recurrence after resection of the primary lesion depends on the stage. The overall recurrence rate ranges from 9% in stage 1–56% in stage 3 CRC tumors [3].

A majority of CRC metastases (mCRC) occurs within the first 3 years. The incidence of mCRC is approximately 4.3% at 1 year, 8.7% at 2 years, 12% at

3 years, and 16.5% at 5 years after resection [2]. The frequency of metachronous CRC metastases is highly variable in the literature, arising from database differences and diversity of definitions. Metachronous CRC metastases are restricted to the liver in 44% of patients with distant recurrence following potentially curative resection of the primary lesion. In prospective and retrospective studies of referral centers, this rate reaches 35% [4]. In prospective observational studies and population studies, this frequency is lower, ranging from 5.7 to 16.3% [5]. In population studies, the frequency of synchronous liver metastases from CRC varies from 14.5 to 24% [2]. Patients presenting with stage 4 disease at the time of the diagnosis will have liver-confined metastases (synchronous metastases) in 77% of the cases [6].

Recently, the clinical outcome for patients with mCRC has improved. Nowadays, the median overall survival (OS) for patients with mCRC is approximately 30 months, more than twice of that observed 20 years ago [7]. It is not clear which improvements and/or strategic changes in the treatment and management of patients with mCRC in recent years have been responsible for the improved treatment outcomes for these patients. Some changes that might have contributed for this gain in OS are (i) changes in the clinical presentation of patients, before the commencement of treatment, due to closer follow-up after resection of the primary tumor and earlier detection of metastatic disease; (ii) improvements in the efficacy of systemic therapies in terms of regimens used, sequence of administration, number of lines of therapy administered, and biomarker-based patient selection; (iii) an increase in the number of patients being treated with a view to facilitating resection of their metastases, offering an increased number of patients the chance of cure and/or durable relapse-free survival and, more recently, the utilization of other ablative therapy techniques with the aim of achieving the same outcome; and (iv) implementation of "continuum of care" treatment strategies coupled with the early integration of optimal supportive care measures [7].

The best treatment strategies for patients with mCRC are evolving rapidly. Superior clinical outcomes are reached when the treatment approaches for individual patients are discussed within a multidisciplinary team (MDT) of experts, meeting regularly as a tumor board to review mCRC cases [8]. The responsibility of the MDT is to define the initial diagnostic workup and then the treatment focus, based on the best diagnostic and therapeutic decision-making available. Initially, the MDT member should critically define whether or not a patient has clearly resectable or initially unresectable metastatic disease. Contrariwise, for patients whose disease is believed "never to be resectable," the discussion may be left to the treating medical oncologist (after discussion with the MDT) and patient as to the pros and cons of various approaches and sequences based on the perceived aims (e.g., duration of disease control versus quality of life and toxicity profiles, etc.) [7].

2. Imaging

The preferred method for the diagnosis of extrahepatic disease is computed tomography (CT) [9–11]. It is the method of choice for staging and follow-up of patients with colorectal cancer, as imaging methods are widespread in our environment, familiar to oncologists, radiologists, and surgeons, with good cost/benefit. Therefore, the use of CT is recommended as the initial method in the diagnosis of extrahepatic metastases.

Magnetic resonance imaging (MRI) is the most accurate imaging technique for the detection and characterization of focal liver lesions. However, costs are higher and it has restricted availability. Other limitations include magnetic field exposure and gadolinium use restrictions in patients with renal insufficiency. Retrospective and meta-analyses have shown that MRI has a superior sensitivity to TC both in analysis per patient (81.1–88.2% vs. 74.8–83.6%) and in analysis per lesion (80.3–86.3% vs. 74.4–82.6%); such superiority is related to higher detection of lesions smaller than 1 cm [12, 13]. MRI with hepatobiliary contrast has demonstrated to have greater accuracy than FDG-PET/CT in detection of small liver metastases (92 vs. 60%) [14]. In a multicenter randomized prospective study, the performance of MRI with hepatobiliary contrast was superior to CT with iodinated contrast and MRI with extracellular gadolinium as first-line method in the initial evaluation of liver mCRC [14].

PET/CT have shown to be of great value in the evaluation of extrahepatic sites of metastases undetected by other methods in patients eligible for surgical resection of liver mCRC, altering the therapeutic plan [15, 16].

Since cross-sectional imaging modalities have improved sensitivity of the diagnosis of mCRC, diagnostic laparoscopy is no longer standard for evaluating patients with mCRC. Instead, it is only used in patients with a suspicion of small-volume carcinomatosis on radiographic imaging studies or who are at particularly high risk for harboring unresectable diseases [17].

3. Prognostic determinants

The pathologic stage at presentation is the most important indicator of outcome after treatment in general, followed by the presence of extramural tumor deposits, lymphovascular and perineural invasion, histologic grade of differentiation, the preoperative level of serum carcinoembryonic antigen (CEA), microsatellite instability (MSI), and RAS and BRAF mutations [18, 19].

Microsatellite instability (MSI) status or mismatch repair deficiency (MMR-D) has been the biomarker for adjuvant 5-FU monotherapy and immune checkpoint inhibitor. Hematogenous and lymphogenous metastasis-dominant CRC with high-frequency MSI (MSI-H) are reported to have poor prognosis. However, the validity as the prognostic factor of MMR is still to be confirmed, and it should thus be used cautiously [20, 21].

On the other hand, it is also known that RAS and BRAF mutations are of prognostic and predictive value in mCRC [21]. The pathogenesis of CRC involves the accumulation of genetic and epigenetic modifications within pathways that regulate proliferation, apoptosis, and angiogenesis.

KRAS mutations involving either codon 12 or 13 can be identified in 12–75% of tumors, and they have been individually correlated with a worse prognosis in most studies [22]. BRAF V600E mutations are present in 8–10% of patients, are consistently associated with poor prognosis, and result in possible patient ineligibility for resection of mCRC [23]. Recently, a small single-center cohort study showed that 21 of 52 patients with BRAF V600E mutant who underwent metastasectomy had longer OS (29.1 vs. 22.7 months) and progression-free survival (13.6 vs. 6.2 months) than the non-metastasectomy cohort. The authors concluded that multimodality therapy incorporating metastasectomy for BRAF V600E metastatic CRC should be considered and might be associated with improved OS in selected patients [24]. Meanwhile, BRAF V600E can be a biomarker for selecting the appropriate chemotherapy regimen [21].

Another feature that also appears to affect the prognosis of patients who develop liver metastases is the embryonic origin of the primary colon cancer. In an analysis of 727 patients who were submitted to chemotherapy followed by resection, mCRC from midgut origin (right colon tumors) was associated with worse pathologic response to chemotherapy and worse survival after resection than mCRC from hindgut origin (left/sigmoid colon tumors) [25]. This effect was independent of the RAS mutation status. Primary tumor from right-sided colon might be more prone to recur. Therefore, palliative resection might not be done since these patients showed no benefit from resection [26].

4. Patient selection

The treatment approach for patients with colorectal liver metastases should be focused toward complete resection whenever possible, with both "oncological" (prognostic) and "technical" (surgical) criteria being considered when evaluating patients for surgery [27, 28].

The "technical" definitions of resectable mCRC have evolved over time, with the current consensus proposing that disease should be considered technically resectable as long as complete macroscopic resection is feasible while maintaining at least a 30% future liver remnant (FLR) or a remnant liver to body weight ratio >0.5 (e.g., >350 g of the liver per 70 kg patient) [29]. Nevertheless, not all patients with technically resectable liver-limited metastases benefit from surgery; approximately half of the patients submitted to resection of mCRC will present widespread systemic disease within 3 years of the resection [30].

Prognostic information that predicts a longer disease-free survival (DFS) or a higher probability of cure is provided by the "oncological" criteria. Strong parameters for the oncological criteria are the number of lesions; the presence, or suspicion, of extrahepatic disease; and numerous other criteria used in retrospective studies. Fong et al. proposed a score based on the following parameters: nodal status of primary tumor, disease-free interval from the primary to discovery of the liver metastases of <12 months, number of tumors >1, preoperative CEA level >200 ng/ml, and size of the largest tumor >5 cm (**Table 1**) [31]. Thus, for some patients, neoadjuvant chemotherapy may be a better option than upfront surgery.

In practice, the patients can be categorized, based upon the criteria above, whether or not they are eligible for resection, as proposed by Adam et al. (**Table 2**) [28]. The disease can be categorized as resectable, not optimally resectable, or unresectable. The not optimally resectable disease is defined as difficult to resect for technical reasons (proximity to hepatic vein and portal vein branches) or technically

Survival (%)						
Score	**1 year**	**2 year**	**3 year**	**4 year**	**5 year**	**Median (mo)**
0	93	79	72	60	60	74
1	91	76	66	54	44	51
2	89	73	60	51	40	47
3	86	67	42	25	20	33
4	70	45	38	29	25	20
5	71	45	27	14	14	22

Each risk factor is one point: node-positive primary, disease-free interval <12 months, >1 tumor, size >5 cm, CEA >200 ng/ml.

Table 1.
Clinical risk score for tumor recurrence proposed by Fong et al. [31].

Category	Contraindication
Technical	
1. Absolute	Impossibility of R0 resection and functional residual liver volume preserved (≥ 25–30% liver remnant) Presence of unresectable extrahepatic disease
2. Relative	R0 resection possible only with complex procedure (portal vein embolization, two-stage hepatectomy, hepatectomy combined with ablation[a]) R1 resection
Oncological	
1.	Concomitant extrahepatic disease (unresectable)
2.	Number of lesion ≥5
3.	Tumor progression

Any patient should be categorized as A1 or A2/B1, B2, or B3. This classification may help to clearly define the type of unresectable patients included in all clinical trials.
[a]Includes all methods, including radiofrequency ablation.

Table 2.
Contraindications to hepatic resection in patients with CRC liver metastases (adapted from Adam et al. [28]).

possible to resect, but oncologically problematic (number of liver metastases greater than 4, maximum diameter 5 cm or more, synchronous liver metastases, primary lymph node metastasis positive, and high levels of tumor markers) [32].

5. Treatment options

Considering the fact that nearly 80% of patients with mCRC are not candidates for resection at diagnosis [33], initial treatment options include chemotherapy and several locoregional therapies. In these cases, chemotherapy in combination with molecular targeted drugs is recommended, followed by curative resection if a response is achieved.

5.1 Chemotherapy

In patients with "favorable oncological" criteria (i.e., >50% likelihood of cure based on various factors including long-term metachronous disease) and "favorable surgical" criteria (no massive disease infiltration), both upfront surgery and perioperative chemotherapy are options. The EPOC study with perioperative chemotherapy has shown no clear predilection for one option over the other, since the 5-year OS rate reported for the perioperative chemotherapy group was 51% (95% CI 45–58) versus 48% (95% CI 40–55) in the surgery-only group [34].

However, in cases with disease that is not technically challenging to resect but where the prognostic situation is unclear, perioperative chemotherapy should be the preferable treatment strategy. These patients should undergo perioperative chemotherapy, 3 months before surgery and 3 months after surgery. The preferred treatment in this situation should be FOLFOX (or alternatively capecitabine with oxaliplatin—CAPOX) as reported for the EPOC trial [34]. EGFR-targeting monoclonal antibodies (cetuximab and panitumumab) are not to be used in this setting, based on the data from the New EPOC trial [35]. No data with bevacizumab are available for this specific patient group; thus, bevacizumab is not indicated [7]. Hence, especially in the case of synchronous metastatic disease, neoadjuvant chemotherapy preceding liver resection is often undertaken as a way of assessing the natural history of metastatic disease prior to resection.

The use of conversion chemotherapy in clinical practice is based on the fact that initially unresectable tumors that are judged resectable after responding to chemotherapy and that undergo surgery display better long-term result than those treated with chemotherapy only [7, 36]. It is reported that up to 33% of patients with "initially unresectable" hepatic metastases have a sufficient objective response to conversion therapy to permit a subsequent complete (R0) resection [17, 37]. However, it has also been reported that the probability of downstaging a truly unresectable disease to the point of resectability is only up to 15 [38].

Another important aspect that has to be studied when considering conversion therapy is that longer durations of chemotherapy increase the possibility of liver toxicity and postoperative complications. Evaluation of the response through imaging tests should be made each 6–8-week gap, and the resection should be made as soon as the metastases are considered undoubtedly resectable [38].

In this scenario the response of the disease to the systemic treatment is also very important. If a growth of the disease is perceived while on chemotherapy or even the development of extrahepatic disease appears in this period, it may indicate that the tumor is biologically aggressive and it would not benefit from resection [17].

After complete resection of mCRC, the best postoperative strategy is debatable as well. Due to the lack of published randomized trials to conduct clinical practice, some suggest completion of a 6-month course of systemic chemotherapy (including courses administered as neoadjuvant therapy), as also suggested by updated guidelines from the National Comprehensive Cancer Network (NCCN) [38].

The strong tumor responses for mCRC with the new agents in chemotherapy can even reach a complete response status. The tumors with less than 2 cm in diameter and more than 1 cm deep in the hepatic parenchyma are the ones with greater risk of vanishing [39]. Nevertheless, the resection is still needed considering that true pathologic complete response or clinical long-term response is, after chemotherapy alone, present in only 17% of the patients [40]. Therefore, those at risk of disappearing with the neoadjuvant treatment should be marked with a fiducial marker such as a coil before chemotherapy [41].

5.2 Radiofrequency ablation therapy

Though resection is considered the gold standard care of mCRC, sometimes there are contraindications due to anatomical reasons. Additionally, there may be comorbidities or liver dysfunction associated which grades the patient as ineligible for major surgery. In these cases, radiofrequency ablation (RFA) represents a great alternative [21].

Considered as a parenchymal-sparing approach, the ablation therapy has been used for managing tumors that can vary from small to unresectable. It can be used as part of a combined ablation/resection tactic in cases of borderline resectable tumors or cases with risk of insufficient future liver remnant [17]. In a multicenter study of 288 patients who underwent combined intraoperative ablation and resection of mCRC, the 5-year overall survival was 37%, and local recurrence-free survival from ablated lesions was 78%. Postoperative mortality was 1%, and the overall complication rate was 35% [42].

5.3 ALPPS

Associating liver partition and portal vein ligation for staged hepatectomy (ALPPS) has emerged as modification on classic two-staged hepatectomy (TSH) with portal vein embolization. This new concept of liver resection, ALPPS, was first described in 2011 [43]. The main advantage of ALPPS is its ability to generate extensive and accelerated hypertrophy of the future liver remnant (FLR), achieving adequate volume for completion of the second stage of the ALPPS in as short as 1 week. This method for hepatic resection has also been described to treat various hepatic tumors in children [44]. ALPPS brings solution to a major flaw of classic TSH, where a considerable percentage (≈30%) of patients are unable to complete the second stage due to insufficient future liver remnant (FLR) growth and short-interval progression of the disease [45].

In the initial study, 68% of the patients experienced complications, and the surgical mortality rate was 12% [43]. Since the first description of ALPPS, there has been a great deal of interest in this treatment. However, criticism of the approach has been raised mainly regarding surgical morbidity and mortality [46].

Recently, Wanis et al. [47] reported a cohort of 58 patients who underwent ALPPS for colorectal liver metastases. They observed no perioperative mortalities and a rate of severe complications of 21%. The 3-year post-ALPPS overall survival was 50%, while the disease-free survival was 13%. The most common site of first recurrence was the liver alone (38%). Patient-reported quality of life after ALPPS was similar to reference values for general population

Additionally, the Scandinavian Multicenter Randomized Controlled Trial (LIGRO Trial) comparing ALPPS with TSH [48], showed a much higher resection rate for ALPPS, 92% (44/48), than TSH, 57% (28/49) ($P < 0.0001$). Considering other parameters, such as complications [43% (19/44) vs. 43% (12/28)] and 90-day mortality [8.3% (4/48) vs. 6.1% (3/49)] or R0 RRs [77% (34/44) vs. 57% (16/28)], no differences were observed.

In experienced hepatobiliary centers and in well-selected patients, ALPPS can be performed with low perioperative morbidity and minimal to no mortality, resulting in good intermediate-term survival and excellent quality of life [47].

Although many centers have been using ALPPS associated with right hepatectomy with good results to treat liver mCRC, indications for ALPPS should continue to be scrutinized critically by multidisciplinary tumor boards based on accepted criteria of remnant liver volume, number of prior cycles of chemotherapy, and histologic criteria of the presence or absence of underlying parenchymal hepatic damage based on at the least a fresh frozen section during stage 1, when considering ALPPS [49].

The technique consists of a bilateral subcostal laparotomy using an adult subcostal retractor. A thorough inspection of the abdominal cavity is carried out in order to detect any previously missed metastases. A cholecystectomy and hepatic hilum dissection are then performed. The right and left hepatic arteries, as well as the arteries for segment 4, were dissected and identified. The common bile duct was dissected. The left or right portal vein is ligated. When the tumor is located on the right hemi-liver with involvement of segment 4, the portal branch for segment 4 is ligated and divided. Full mobilization of the liver is obtained by sectioning the falciform, coronary, and right and left triangular ligaments of the liver. The right or left hepatic vein of the liver to be resected is dissected and encircled with a vessel loop, as seen in **Figure 1**. An intraoperative ultrasound is performed to verify a tumor-free parenchymal transection line.

The liver parenchyma is transected using combined ultrasonic energy (Ultracision®), monopolar and bipolar electrocautery, and ligation of the blood vessels and bile ducts. Biologic fibrin sealant can be used in both surfaces of the spitted liver. Closed drainage is placed in the liver hilum. We do not use any plastic film, mesh, or plastic bag to separate both surfaces of the liver. Metastases located in the future remnant liver (FRL) can be treated either by local resection or radiofrequency tumor ablation (RFA).

During the second operation, the hepatic artery and the bile duct of the diseased liver are ligated and transected. A clamp is applied at the right or left hepatic vein,

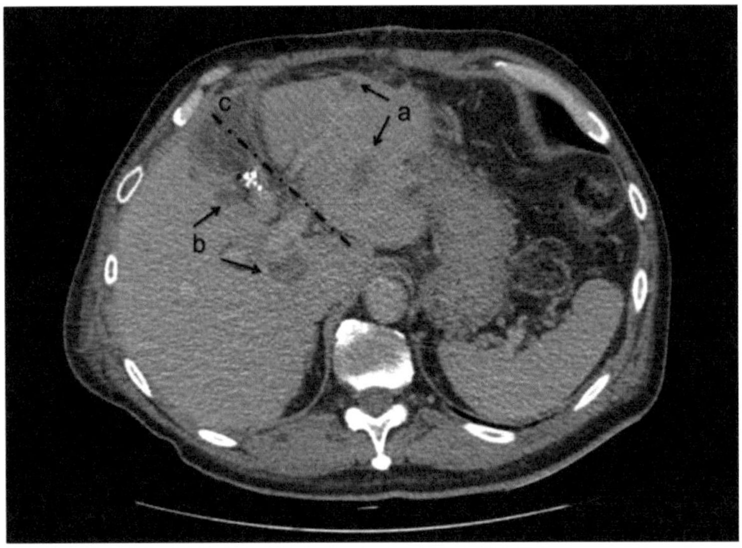

Figure 1.
Postoperative CT image of a patient who underwent portal vein ligation and staged hepatectomy: (a) treated liver metastases of the FRL, (b) metastases on liver to be resected, and (c) line of liver bipartition.

and the vein is then transected. A 4–0 Prolene® running suture is applied to the stump of the hepatic vein. Liver segment 1 is usually preserved [46].

6. Timing for surgical approach

When facing a situation of synchronous disease, with both primary tumor and hepatic metastases, the timing for surgical approach of the hepatic lesions is still a topic of discussion.

The lesions can be accessed simultaneously in one procedure, or they can be treated with a staged resection. In the staged manner, there is the classic approach, which means accessing the primary tumor first; and there is the reverse approach, also known as liver-first approach. No difference has been shown by various studies, regardless of which method is used [50].

Therefore, the decision should be established on a case-by-case basis, considering the symptoms presented by the patient, location, size, and possible complications of each one such as bowel perforation, risk of liver failure, whether the patient underwent chemotherapy or not, performance status, and the surgeon expertise [17, 51].

7. Surgical resection

The surgical approach of the mCRC in the liver can be performed through an anatomic resection or a nonanatomic/parenchymal-sparing resection (PSR). Since the type of resection has not been associated with significant differences in rates of positive margin, recurrence, or survival [50], and considering that the PSR preserves greater hepatic reserve, recent studies are leaning toward the nonanatomic method, particularly when chemotherapy-induced liver injury is a concern [17].

Keeping in mind that recurrences after initial resection of mCRC can occur in up to 57% of cases and the most common site of recurrences is the liver [52] and considering that repeat liver resection in a second recurrence, with satisfactory morbidity and perioperative mortality, has been associated with a 5-year survival up to 43% [38], the PSR becomes an even more attractive option.

Considering the width of the resection margin, a 2017 meta-analysis reported that margins greater than 10 mm were related with superior 5-year OS [53]. Still, numerous retrospective studies revealed that less than 10 mm but negative margin is not related with poorer survival [54]. In a multicenter study of 551 patients, surgical margins were classified as positive or negative with 1–4, 5–9, and >10 mm of tumor-free parenchyma. The positive margins were associated with a greater risk of recurrence, and the width of negative margins did not affect survival, recurrence, or site of recurrences [54].

There is one situation where anatomic resection and/or a wider surgical margin (>10 mm) may be indicated which is before a RAS-mutated mCRC as it constitutes a more aggressive tumor biology group and has been associated with more positive margins and worse survival after surgery [55]. Others reported that even a wider resection margin might not be sufficient to overcome the aggressive tumor biology associated with a RAS mutation. In a study of 411 patients who underwent resection for mCRC at Johns Hopkins University, a 1–4-mm margin was associated with improved survival compared with a positive margin (<1 mm or R1) for wild-type KRAS tumors, with which a wider resection margin did not further improve survival. In KRAS-mutated tumors, however, negative margin status, which included a 1-cm margin, did not improve survival [56].

8. Follow-up after resection

According to the consensus-based guidelines from the National Comprehensive Cancer Network (NCCN), the recommendation is carcinoembryonic antigen (CEA) testing every 3–6 months for 2 years followed by every 6 months for 3 years; computed tomography (CT) of the chest/abdomen and pelvis every 3–6 months for 2 years and then every 6–12 months up to a total of 5 years; colonoscopy in 1 year; if negative, repeat in 3 years and then every 5 years; and if advanced adenoma is found, repeat in 1 year [38].

An important point is that posttreatment follow-up should only be performed for those patients considered candidate for a second potentially curative surgical procedure [38].

9. Repeat resection for colorectal liver metastases

Re-resection for recurrence of mCRC is a safe and viable option in properly selected patients. In order to prevent post-hepatectomy liver failure, sufficient future liver reserve is paramount, as well as no evidence of extrahepatic disease and good performance status [57–59].

Although randomized trials have not been conducted to prove benefit, several reported series have demonstrated perioperative mortality rates lower than 5%, and overall survival rates ranged from 20 to 43% at 2–5 years [57–59].

Patients with a relapse-free interval of longer than 1 year appear to have a more favorable outcome from re-resection. Factors associated with a poor outcome include synchronous resection for the first liver metastases and the presence of multiple lesions at second hepatectomy [60, 61].

Interestingly, recurrences at the margin are uncommon [62, 63]. Some studies have reported 5-year overall survival rates after re-resection of 33–73% with no perioperative mortality [64, 65].

10. Conclusion

It is known that the majority of metastatic CRC liver disease will be potentially resectable at the time of diagnosis. Considering that hepatic resection is the only curative option for these patients, the parameters of resectability have expanded through the years due to a wider knowledge of the disease, improving diagnostic techniques, new drugs, and technical surgical advances. It is safe to say that the treatment strategies have advanced rapidly enough to change dramatically the natural history of the mCRC.

ALPPS has been recently introduced as an option to the treatment of mCRC. It has been shown to increase drastically the resection rates, with complications rates not different from standard two-staged hepatectomy.

Several treatment options are available to treat patients with mCRC. It is important to have in mind that the treatment approach must be established for each case. Not only the patient and anatomic factors are important, but also the tumor factors must be considered. Best results are obtained when the treatment approaches for individual patients are discussed within a multidisciplinary team (MDT) of experts, meeting regularly as a tumor board to review mCRC cases.

Author details

Julio Wiederkehr*, Barbara Wiederkehr and Henrique Wiederkehr
Federal University of Parana, Curitiba, Brazil

*Address all correspondence to: julio.wieder@gmail.com

References

[1] Ferlay J, Soerjomataram I, Dikshit R, Eser S, Mathers C, Rebelo M, et al. Cancer incidence and mortality worldwide: Sources, methods and major patterns in GLOBOCAN 2012. International Journal of Cancer. 2015;**136**(5):E359-E386

[2] Coimbra FJF, Ribeiro HS, Marques MC, Herman P, Chojniak R, Kalil AN, et al. First brazilian consensus on multimodal treatment of colorectal liver metastases. Module 1: Pre-treatment evaluation. ABCD Arquivos Brasileiros de Cirurgia Digestiva (São Paulo). 2015;**28**(4):222-230 Available from: http://www.scielo.br/scielo.php?script=sci_arttext&pid=S0102-67202015000400222&lng=en&nrm=iso&tlng=en

[3] Siegel R, Ward E, Brawley O, Jemal A. Cancer statistics, 2011: The impact of eliminating socioeconomic and racial disparities on premature cancer deaths. CA: S Cancer Journal for Clinicians. 2011;**61**:212-236

[4] Thomasset SC, Dennison AR, Metcalfe MS, Steward WP, Garcea G. Changing trends in the presentation of colorectal liver metastases in a single hepatobiliary tertiary referral centre over fourteen years. European Journal of Surgical Oncology, Elsevier Ltd. 2013;**39**(11):1243-1247 Available from: http://dx.doi.org/10.1016/j.ejso.2013.08.021

[5] Manfredi S, Lepage C, Hatem C, Coatmeur O, Faivre J, Bouvier AM. Epidemiology and management of liver metastases from colorectal cancer. Annals of Surgery. 2006;**244**(2):254-259

[6] Alberts SR. Update on the optimal management of patients with colorectal liver metastases. Critical Reviews in Oncology/Hematology, Elsevier Ireland Ltd. 2012;**84**(1):59-70. Available from: http://dx.doi.org/10.1016/j.critrevonc.2012.02.007

[7] Van Cutsem E, Cervantes A, Adam R, Sobrero A, Van Krieken JH, Aderka D, et al. ESMO consensus guidelines for the management of patients with metastatic colorectal cancer. Annals of Oncology. 2016;**27**(8):1386-1422

[8] Shah S, Arora S, Atkin G, Glynne-Jones R, Mathur P, Darzi A, et al. Decision-making in Colorectal Cancer Tumor Board meetings: Results of a prospective observational assessment. Surgical Endoscopy. 2014;**28**(10):2783-2788

[9] Fowler KJ, Linehan DC, Menias CO. Colorectal liver metastases: State of the art imaging. Annals of Surgical Oncology. 2013;**20**(4):1185-1193

[10] Kekelidze M, D'Errico L, Pansini M, Tyndall A, Hohmann J. Colorectal cancer: Current imaging methods and future perspectives for the diagnosis, staging and therapeutic response evaluation. World Journal of Gastroenterology. 2013;**19**(46):8502-8514

[11] Tudyka V, Blomqvist L, Beets-Tan RGH, Boelens PG, Valentini V, Van De Velde CJ, et al. EURECCA consensus conference highlights about colon & rectal cancer multidisciplinary management: The radiology experts review. European Journal of Surgical Oncology, Elsevier Ltd. 2014;**40**(4):469-475. Available from: http://dx.doi.org/10.1016/j.ejso.2013.10.029

[12] Shimada K, Isoda H, Hirokawa Y, Arizono S, Shibata T, Togashi K. Comparison of gadolinium-EOB-DTPA-enhanced and diffusion-weighted liver MRI for detection of small hepatic metastases. European Radiology. 2010;**20**(11):2690-2698

[13] Koh D-M, Collins DJ, Wallace T, Chau I, Riddell AM. Combining diffusion-weighted MRI with Gd-EOB-DTPA-enhanced MRI improves the detection of colorectal liver metastases. British Journal of Radiology. 2012;**85**(1015):980-989. Available from: http://www.birpublications.org/doi/10.1259/bjr/91771639

[14] Moulton CA, Gu CS, Law CH, Tandan VR, Hart R, Quan D, et al. Effect of PET before liver resection on surgical management for colorectal adenocarcinoma metastases. Journal of the American Medical Association. 2014;**311**(18):1863. Available from: http://jama.jamanetwork.com/article.aspx?doi=10.1001/jama.2014.3740

[15] Chun YS, Vauthey J-N, Boonsirikamchai P, Maru DM, Kopetz S, Palavecino M, et al. Association of computed tomography morphologic criteria with pathologic response and survival in patients treated with bevacizumab for colorectal liver metastases. Journal of the American Medical Association. 2009;**302**(21):2338-2344. Available from: http://www.pubmedcentral.nih.gov/articlerender.fcgi?artid=4139149&tool=pmcentrez&rendertype=abstract

[16] Figueiras RG, Goh V, Padhani AR, Naveira AB, Caamaño AG, Martin CV. The role of functional imaging in colorectal cancer. American Journal of Roentgenology. 2010;**195**(1):54-66

[17] Hepatic Resection for Colorectal Cancer Liver Metastasis–UpToDate [Cited July 9]. 2018. Available from: https://www.uptodate.com/contents/hepatic-resection-for-colorectal-cancer-liver-metastasis?search=cancer colorretal LIVER&source=search_result&selectedTitle=3~150&usage_type=default&display_rank=3

[18] Edge SB, Byrd DR, Compton CC, et al., editors. AJCC (American Joint Committee on Cancer) Cancer Staging Manual. 7th ed. New York: Springer; 2010. p. 133. no abstract available. [cited 2018 Jul 10]. Available from: https://www.uptodate.com/contents/pathology-and-prognostic-determinants-of-colorectal-cancer/abstract/29

[19] Pathology and Prognostic Determinants of Colorectal Cancer–UpToDate [cited Jul 10]. 2018. Available from: https://www.uptodate.com/contents/pathology-and-prognostic-determinants-of-colorectal-cancer?sectionName=RAS and BRAF&topicRef=115954&anchor=H1022797966&source=see_link#H1022797966

[20] Fujiyoshi K, Yamamoto G, Takenoya T, et al. Metastatic pattern of stage IV colorectal cancer with high-frequency microsatellite instability as a prognostic factor. Anticancer Research. 2017;**37**:239-247

[21] Oki E, Ando K, Nakanishi R, Sugiyama M, Nakashima Y, Kubo N, et al. Recent advances in treatment for colorectal liver metastasis. Annals of Gastroenterological Surgery. 2018;**2**:167-175

[22] Modest DP, Ricard I, Heinemann V, Hegewisch-Becker S, Schmiegel W, Porschen R, et al. Outcome according to KRAS-, NRAS- and BRAF-mutation as well as KRAS mutation variants: Pooled analysis of five randomized trials in metastatic colorectal cancer by the AIO colorectal cancer study group. Annals of Oncology: An Official Journal of the European Society for Medical Oncology. 2016;**27**(9):1746-1753. Available from: https://academic.oup.com/annonc/article-lookup/doi/10.1093/annonc/mdw261

[23] Passiglia F, Bronte G, Bazan V, Galvano A, Vincenzi BRA. Can KRAS and BRAF mutations limit the benefit of liver resection in metastatic colorectal cancer patients? A systematic review and meta-analysis. Critical Reviews in Oncology/Hematology. 2016;**99**:150-157

[24] Johnson B, Jin Z, Truty MJ, et al. Impact of metastasectomy in the multimodality approach for BRAF V600E metastatic colorectal cancer: The Mayo Clinic experience. The Oncologist. 2018;**23**(1):128-134

[25] Yamashita S, Brudvik KW, Kopetz SE, Maru D, Clarke CN, Passot G, et al. Embryonic origin of primary colon cancer predicts pathologic response and survival in patients undergoing resection for colon cancer liver metastases. Annals of Surgery, NIH Public Access. 2018;**267**(3):514-520. Available from: http://www.ncbi.nlm.nih.gov/pubmed/28002060

[26] Zhang RX, Ma WJ, Gu YT, et al. Primary tumor location as a predictor of the benefit of palliative resection for colorectal cancer with unresectable metastasis. World Journal of Surgical Oncology. 2017;**15**(1):138

[27] Aloia TA, Adam R, Azoulay D, et al. Outcome following hepatic resection of metastatic renal tumors: The Paul Brousse Hospital experience. Oxford: HPB; 2006;**8**(2):100-105

[28] Adam R, De Gramont A, Figueras J, Guthrie A, Kokudo N, Kunstlinger F, et al. The oncosurgery approach to managing liver metastases from colorectal cancer: A multidisciplinary international consensus. The Oncologist. 2012;**17**(10):1225-1239

[29] Clavien PA, Petrowsky H, DeOliveira ML, Graf R. Strategies for safer liver surgery and partial liver transplantation. The New England Journal of Medicine. 2007;**356**(15):1545-1559. Available from: http://www.nejm.org/doi/abs/10.1056/NEJMra065156

[30] Kanas GP, Taylor A, Primrose JN, Langeberg WJ, Kelsh MA, Mowat FS, et al. Survival after liver resection in metastatic colorectal cancer: Review and meta-analysis of prognostic factors. Clinical Epidemiology. 2012;**4**(1):283-301

[31] Fong Y, Fortner J, Sun RL, et al. Clinical score for predicting recurrence after hepatic resection for metastatic colorectal cancer: Analysis of 1001 consecutive cases. Annals of Surgery. 1999;**230**(3):309-321

[32] Nordlinger B, Van Cutsem E, Gruenberger T, Glimelius B, Poston G, Rougie P, et al. Combination of surgery and chemotherapy and the role of targeted agents in the treatment of patients with colorectal liver metastases: Recommendations from an expert panel. Annals of Oncology. 2009;**20**(6):985-992

[33] Garden OJ, Rees M, Poston GJ, Mirza D, Saunders M, Ledermann J, et al. Guidelines for resection of colorectal cancer liver metastases. Gut. 2006;**55**(Suppl 3):iii1-iii8. Available from: http://gut.bmj.com/cgi/doi/10.1136/gut.2006.098053

[34] Nordlinger B, Sorbye H, Glimelius B, Poston GJ, Schlag PM, Rougier P, et al. Perioperative FOLFOX4 chemotherapy and surgery versus surgery alone for resectable liver metastases from colorectal cancer (EORTC 40983): Long-term results of a randomised, controlled, phase 3 trial. The Lancet Oncology. 2013;**14**(12):1208-1215

[35] Primrose J, Falk S, Finch-Jones M, Valle J, O'Reilly D, Siriwardena A, et al. Systemic chemotherapy with or without cetuximab in patients with resectable colorectal liver metastasis: The New EPOC randomised controlled trial. The Lancet Oncology. 2014;**15**(6):601-611

[36] Adam R, Bhangui P, Poston G, Mirza D, Nuzzo G, Barroso E, et al. Is perioperative chemotherapy useful for solitary, metachronous, colorectal liver metastases? Annals of Surgery. 2010;**252**(5):774-785

[37] Barone C, Nuzzo G, Cassano A, Basso M, Schinzari G, Giuliante F, et al.

Final analysis of colorectal cancer patients treated with irinotecan and 5-fluorouracil plus folinic acid neoadjuvant chemotherapy for unresectable liver metastases. British Journal of Cancer. 2007;**97**(8):1035-1039. Available from: http://www.nature.com/articles/6603988

[38] Management of Potentially Resectable Colorectal Cancer Liver Metastases–UpToDate [cited Jul 11]. 2018. Available from: https://www.uptodate.com/contents/management-of-potentially-resectable-colorectal-cancer-liver-metastases?search=cancer colorretal LIVER&source=search_result&selectedTitle=1~150&usage_type=default&display_rank=1

[39] Passot G, Odisio BC, Zorzi D, Mahvash A, Gupta S, Wallace MJ, et al. Eradication of missing liver metastases after fiducial placement. Journal of Gastrointestinal Surgery. 2016;**20**(6):1173-1178. Available from: http://link.springer.com/10.1007/s11605-016-3079-1

[40] Benoist S, Brouquet A, Penna C, Julié C, El Hajjam M, Chagnon S, et al. Complete response of colorectal liver metastases after chemotherapy: Does it mean cure? Journal of Clinical Oncology. 2006;**24**(24):3939-3945. Available from: http://ascopubs.org/doi/10.1200/JCO.2006.05.8727

[41] Zalinski S, Abdalla EK, Mahvash A, Vauthey JN. A marking technique for intraoperative localization of small liver metastases before systemic chemotherapy. Annals of Surgical Oncology. 2009;**16**(5):1208-1211. Available from: http://www.springerlink.com/index/10.1245/s10434-009-0328-5

[42] Evrard S, Poston G, Kissmeyer-Nielsen P, Diallo A, Desolneux G, Brouste V, et al. Combined ablation and resection (CARe) as an effective parenchymal sparing treatment for extensive colorectal liver metastases. In: Taketomi A, editor. PLoS One. 2014;**9**(12):e114404. Available from: http://dx.plos.org/10.1371/journal.pone.0114404

[43] Schnitzbauer AA, Lang SA, Goessmann H, Nadalin S, Baumgart J, Farkas SA, et al. Right portal vein ligation combined with in situ splitting induces rapid left lateral liver lobe hypertrophy enabling 2-staged extended right hepatic resection in small-for-size settings. Annals of Surgery. 2012;**255**(3):405-414

[44] Wiederkehr JC, Avilla SG, Mattos E, Coelho IM, Ledesma JA, Conceição AF, et al. Associating liver partition with portal vein ligation and staged hepatectomy (ALPPS) for the treatment of liver tumors in children. Journal of Pediatric Surgery. 2015;**50**(7):1227-1231

[45] Lam VWT, Laurence JM, Johnston E, Hollands MJ, Pleass HCC, Richardson AJ. A systematic review of two-stage hepatectomy in patients with initially unresectable colorectal liver metastases. HPB. 2013;**15**(7):483-491

[46] Shindoh J, Vauthey J-N, Zimmitti G, Curley SA, Huang SY, et al. Analysis of the efficacy of portal vein embolization for patients with extensive liver malignancy and very low future liver remnant volume, including a comparison with the associating liver partition with portal vein ligation for staged hepatectomy approach. Journal of American College of Surgeons. Jul 2013;**217**(1):126-134. DOI: 10.1016/j.jamcollsurg.2013.03.004. Epub 2013 Apr 28

[47] Wanis KN, Ardiles V, Alvarez FA, Tun-Abraham ME, Linehan D, de Santibañes E, et al. Intermediate-term survival and quality of life outcomes in patients with advanced colorectal liver metastases undergoing associating liver partition and portal vein ligation for staged hepatectomy. Surgery (United States), Elsevier Inc., Available from. 2018;**163**(4):691-697

https://doi.org/10.1016/j.surg.2017.09.044

[48] Sandström P, Røsok BI, Sparrelid E, Larsen PN, Larsson AL, Lindell G, et al. ALPPS improves resectability compared with conventional two-stage hepatectomy in patients with advanced colorectal liver metastasis: Results from a scandinavian multicenter randomized controlled trial (LIGRO trial). Annals of Surgery. 2018;**267**(5):833-840

[49] Schnitzbauer AA, Schadde E, Linecker M, Machado MA, Adam R, Malago M, et al. Indicating ALPPS for colorectal liver metastases: A critical analysis of patients in the international ALPPS registry. Surgery (United States), Elsevier Inc.; 2018;**164**(3):387-394. Available from: https://doi.org/10.1016/j.surg.2018.02.026

[50] Sarpel U, Bonavia AS, Grucela A, Roayaie S, Schwartz ME, Labow DM. Does anatomic versus nonanatomic resection affect recurrence and survival in patients undergoing surgery for colorectal liver metastasis? Annals of Surgical Oncology. 2009;**16**(2):379-384. Available from: http://www.springerlink.com/index/10.1245/s10434-008-0218-2

[51] Veereman G, Robays J, Verleye L, Leroy R, Rolfo C, Van Cutsem E, et al. Pooled analysis of the surgical treatment for colorectal cancer liver metastases. Critical Reviews in Oncology/Hematology. 2015;**94**(1):122-135. Available from: http://linkinghub.elsevier.com/retrieve/pii/S1040842814002121

[52] De Jong MC, Pulitano C, Ribero D, Strub J, Mentha G, Schulick RD, et al. Rates and patterns of recurrence following curative intent surgery for colorectal liver metastasis: An international multi-institutional analysis of 1669 patients. Annals of Surgery. 2009;**250**(3):440-447

[53] Margonis GA, Sergentanis TN, Ntanasis-Stathopoulos I, Andreatos N, Tzanninis I-G, Sasaki K, et al. Impact of surgical margin width on recurrence and overall survival following R0 hepatic resection of colorectal metastases: A systematic review and meta-analysis. Annals of Surgery. 2018;**267**(6):1047-1055. Available from: http://insights.ovid.com/crossref?an=00000658-201806000-00012

[54] Pawlik TM, Scoggins CR, Zorzi D, Abdalla EK, Andres A, Eng C, et al. Effect of surgical margin status on survival and site of recurrence after hepatic resection for colorectal metastases. Annals of Surgery. 2005;**241**(5):715-722, discussion 722-4. Available from http://www.ncbi.nlm.nih.gov/pubmed/15849507

[55] Brudvik KW, Mise Y, Chung MH, Chun YS, Kopetz SE, Passot G, et al. RAS mutation predicts positive resection margins and narrower resection margins in patients undergoing resection of colorectal liver metastases. Annals of Surgical Oncology. 2016;**23**(8):2635-2643. Available from: http://link.springer.com/10.1245/s10434-016-5187-2

[56] Margonis GA, Sasaki K, Andreatos N, Kim Y, Merath K, Wagner D, et al. KRAS mutation status dictates optimal surgical margin width in patients undergoing resection of colorectal liver metastases. Annals of Surgical Oncology. 2017;**24**(1):264-271. Available from: http://link.springer.com/10.1245/s10434-016-5609-1

[57] Butte JM, Gönen M, Allen PJ, Peter Kingham T, Sofocleous CT, DeMatteo RP, et al. Recurrence after partial hepatectomy for metastatic colorectal cancer: Potentially curative role of salvage repeat resection. Annals of Surgical Oncology. 2015;**22**(8):2761-2771. Available from: http://link.springer.com/10.1245/s10434-015-4370-1

[58] Wicherts DA, de Haas RJ, Salloum C, Andreani P, Pascal G, Sotirov D,

et al. Repeat hepatectomy for recurrent colorectal metastases. British Journal of Surgery. 2013;**100**(6):808-818. Available from: http://doi.wiley.com/10.1002/bjs.9088

[59] Adair RA, Young AL, Cockbain AJ, Malde D, Prasad KR, Lodge JPA, et al. Repeat hepatic resection for colorectal liver metastases. British Journal of Surgery. 2012;**99**(9):1278-1283. Available from: http://doi.wiley.com/10.1002/bjs.8845

[60] Ishiguro S, Akasu T, Fujimoto Y, Yamamoto J, Sakamoto Y, Sano T, et al. Second hepatectomy for recurrent colorectal liver metastasis: Analysis of preoperative prognostic factors. Annals of Surgical Oncology. 2006;**13**(12):1579-1587. Available from: http://www.springerlink.com/index/10.1245/s10434-006-9067-z

[61] Gomez D, Sangha VK, Morris-Stiff G, Malik HZ, Guthrie AJ, Toogood GJ, et al. Outcomes of intensive surveillance after resection of hepatic colorectal metastases. British Journal of Surgery. 2010;**97**(10):1552-1560. Available from: http://doi.wiley.com/10.1002/bjs.7136

[62] Bodingbauer M, Tamandl D, Schmid K, Plank C, Schima W, Gruenberger T. Size of surgical margin does not influence recurrence rates after curative liver resection for colorectal cancer liver metastases. British Journal of Surgery. 2007;**94**(9):1133-1138. Available from: http://doi.wiley.com/10.1002/bjs.5762

[63] de Haas RJ, Wicherts DA, Flores E, Azoulay D, Castaing D, Adam R. R1 resection by necessity for colorectal liver metastases: Is it still a contraindication to surgery? Annals of Surgery. 2008;**248**(4):626-637. Available from: https://insights.ovid.com/crossref?an=00153307-200801260-00031

[64] Andreou A, Brouquet A, Abdalla EK, Aloia TA, Curley SA, Vauthey JN. Repeat hepatectomy for recurrent colorectal liver metastases is associated with a high survival rate. HPB (Oxford). 2011;**13**(11):774-782. Available from: http://linkinghub.elsevier.com/retrieve/pii/S1365182X15303749

[65] Neal CP, Nana GR, Jones M, Cairns V, Ngu W, Isherwood J, et al. Repeat hepatectomy is independently associated with favorable long-term outcome in patients with colorectal liver metastases. Cancer Medicine. 2017;**6**(2):331-338. Available from: http://doi.wiley.com/10.1002/cam4.872

Chapter 8

Cholangiocarcinoma

Samuel Romeo Obiekwe, Nathaly Suzett De La Roca and Jean Saric

Abstract

Cholangiocarcinoma is a malignant disease of the biliary ductal system which consists of intrahepatic (periphery) 5–10% and extrahepatic, which is further divided into proximal (perihilar) 60–70% and distal 20–30%. The etiology of this grave disease is unknown although many causative factors, including infectious, congenital, and genetic factors, causing chronic inflammation, which results in dysplastic changes of the biliary epithelium and eventual malignancy, have been implicated. The prognosis is poor except when discovered early. The treatment of intrahepatic (CCA) is partial hepatectomy, while radical bile duct resection with or without hepatectomy or pancreaticoduodenectomy is considered for extrahepatic cancer. Liver transplantation is considered in advanced diseases, without extrahepatic lymph node involvement. Palliation including endoscopic drainage or surgical bypass which is an option for unresectable diseases. Adjuvant therapy in the form of chemotherapy, immunotherapy, and photodynamic therapy is a consideration in patients with advanced disease. Many advances have been made in the treatment of cholangiocarcinoma, and hopefully long-term survival may be improved.

Keywords: bile duct cancer, etiology, treatment, resection, palliation, prognosis

1. Introduction

This grave illness was first described in 1840 by Durand-Fardel, as a malignant neoplasia arising from the epithelial cells of the extrahepatic and intrahepatic bile ducts, excluding the papilla of Vater and gallbladder. In 1965, Gerald Klatskin, a Yale University pathologist, described the adenocarcinoma of porta hepatis. Adenocarcinoma of the bile duct epithelium or cholangiocarcinoma within the confluence of the right and left hepatic duct has since then been known as "Klatskin tumor." The majority of this disease arises at the hepatic duct bifurcation. Surgical resection offers the only chance for cure of this disease. Unfortunately, many patients present with advanced locoregional and distant metastasis at the time of diagnosis, making palliative procedures aimed at biliary drainage with intent to prevent progressive liver failure and cholangitis, which is the only option for unresectable tumors [1–4].

Cholangiocarcinoma (CC) is classified into proximal, perihilar or Klatskin's (60–70%), distal (20–30%), and intrahepatic or periphery (5–10%). They all have different pathophysiological, epidemiological, and clinical presentations. The most important modality of treatment for hilar cholangiocarcinoma is radical bile duct resection with partial hepatectomy and maintenance of bilioenteric continuity. For intrahepatic cholangiocarcinoma, partial hepatectomy is the treatment of choice, whereas distal cholangiocarcinoma may require pancreaticoduodenectomy. Surgical outcome after resection for distal cholangiocarcinoma is superior to the rest. Some subset of highly selected patients with unresectable hilar cholangiocarcinoma (HCCA) or intrahepatic cholangiocarcinoma (ICCA) orthotopic liver transplantation (OLT) may be a viable option and has been reported to provide survival benefits [5, 6].

2. Incidence

Statistics of autopsy report shows that the incidence of bile duct carcinoma is 0.01–0.5%. In the United States, it is 1–100,000 per year, with 3000 new cases diagnosed yearly. Worldwide incidence is 0.5–2.0/100,000. Complete resection of early stage tumors can be curative. When the disease is unresectable, prognosis is generally poor with 1-year survival of 53% and 5-year survival of less than 5%. Bile duct cancer is rare in Western countries, resulting in less than 2% in all human cancers. It varies widely in different parts of the world. For example, in Thailand the incidence is 113/100,000 in men and 50/100,000 in women, whereas in France it is 1.7 and 0.5 per 100,000. In Australia, the incidence is low 0.2/100,000 in men and 0.1/100,000 in women. In the United States, studies have shown a decline from 0.85 per 100,000 in 1995 to 0.58 per 100,000 in 2005. The frequency of bile duct cancer increases with age, the majority of these patients are above 65 years old, with peak incidence at seventh decade of life. Cholangiocarcinoma rarely occurs before the age of 40 except in patients with congenital bile duct cysts. The incidence is higher in men than women with a ratio of 1:(1.2–1.5). In the past three decades, most studies have shown a worldwide increase in the mortality from intrahepatic cholangiocarcinoma, whereas there is a decrease in mortality for extrahepatic and gallbladder cancer [7–9].

3. Causative factors

The etiology of cholangiocarcinoma is unknown; however, several risk factors proven and unproven have been attributed as a causative factor for this grave illness. The cause of cholangiocarcinoma is associated with chronic biliary inflammation; malignant transformation may occur in the background of chronic inflammation and cholestasis. The production of some cytokines and reactive oxygen species may cause permanent damage to the DNA.

4. Risk factors

The established risk factors for cholangiocarcinoma include bile duct cysts, parasitic infection, primary sclerosing cholangitis (PSC), hepatolithiasis, and toxins. Other potential established risk factors include inflammatory bowel disease (IBD), hepatitis B and hepatitis C, liver cirrhosis, diabetes, obesity, alcohol, smoking, and host genetic polymorphisms. Thorotrast, a contrast medium which is no longer in use, although used between 1930 and 1960, was associated with several tumors including primary liver tumor, angiosarcomas, gallbladder carcinomas, and tumors of the extrahepatic bile duct. Several large studies from Japan, Germany, and Denmark showed that 45.6% of the patients exposed to Thorotrast developed liver cancer 15–20 years after exposure, compared to 0.3% of control. This is because biological half-life of Thorotrast is 400 years. As with other tumors, dietary nitrosamines are also implicated [10, 11]. Primary sclerosing cholangitis, an autoimmune disease that results in stricturing of extra- and intrahepatic bile ducts, is an established risk factor for CC. Chronic inflammation, proliferation of biliary epithelium, production of endogenous bile mutagens, and bile stasis are postulated mechanisms of carcinogenesis. About 70% of patients with PSC also suffer from ulcerative colitis, but only a minority of patients with ulcerative colitis develops PSC, so that patients with ulcerative colitis who do not have symptoms of PSC may have increased risk of cholangiocarcinoma. It is interesting that surgical or medical treatment of ulcerative colitis does not decrease the risk of developing cholangiocarcinoma in patients with ulcerative colitis [12]. Hepatobiliary flukes *Opisthorchis viverrini* (*O. vivverini*) and *Clonorchis sinensis* (*C. sinensis*) are associated with cholangiocarcinoma irrespective of site, especially in Southeast Asia. They are trematodes that inhabit in the bile ducts, occasionally the gallbladder, and the pancreatic duct of mammals. Infestation of humans occurs via ingestion of raw, pickled, or undercooked fish. Both parasites increase the susceptibility of cholangiocytes to carcinogens causing chronic irritation and inflammation. Typhoid organisms have been implicated in patients with cholangiocarcinoma, as well as chronic recurrent pyogenic bacterial cholangitis [13, 14].

Hepatolithiasis are stone or gravel located in the intrahepatic biliary tree. Hepatolithiasis is rare in the Western Hemisphere but more common in Southeast Asia notably in Taiwan. These parasitic infestations, such as *Clonorchis sinensis* and *Ascaris lumbricoides*, have been implicated in most patients with hepatolithiasis. Because it is common in Asian countries, it is considered an important risk factor for cholangiocarcinoma. The relationship between hepatolithiasis and cholangiocarcinoma is not well established in the Western Hemisphere, except an Italian study which showed a significant association between hepatolithiasis and ICCA [15, 16]. Patients with congenital biliary disease have an increased risk of developing CC, compared to general population. The risk is highest in patients who did not undergo surgical treatment, who have complete cysts excision before the age of 20, and in those treated with cyst drainage alone, instead of complete cysts excision. There are different types of bile duct cysts, such as extrahepatic biliary cysts and intrahepatic biliary cysts. The etiology of cancer in patients with biliary cysts is as a result of chronic irritation from the reflux of pancreatic enzymes, cholestasis, and damaging effect of bile acids to biliary epithelium, resulting in the formation of malignant cells in patients with bile duct cysts. The average age of cancer formation is around 32, which is younger than the age of presentation of CC in the general population. The risk of malignancy decreases in patients undergoing complete choledochal cyst excision; surprisingly, these patients are still at an increased risk of developing CC than the general population. Patients with an anomalous pancreaticobiliary ductal junction (APBDJ) have a higher incidence of developing bile duct cancer. Ohta showed dysplastic mucosa in this group of patients [17–22].

Tocchi et al. did a retrospective review in patients with biliary-enteric drainage for benign disease and found a high incidence of CC in this population, 5.8% in those who underwent transduodenal sphincteroplasty, 7.6% in choledochoduodenostomy patients, and 1.9% in patients who had undergone hepaticojejunostomy [23].

Bile duct adenomas and multiple biliary papillomatosis have been shown to have malignant transformation potential [24, 25]. Hepatitis C (HCV), hepatitis B (HBV), and liver cirrhosis, regardless of etiology, have been shown as a risk factor for ICCA [26].

There is an association between hepatitis C and cholangiocarcinoma in the United States as reported in Japan. This association is not well studied, but cirrhosis is implicated here [27]. Some studies from the Western countries, such as Denmark, examined a large population of patients with liver cirrhosis over a mean follow-up period of 6 years and showed an increase risk of cholangiocarcinoma in patients with cirrhosis than general population. An Italian study also demonstrated an association between HCV and ICCA [16, 28]. As mentioned above, the Japanese study showed an association between hepatitis C and cholangiocarcinoma. This is not represented in the study from Korea and Thailand, where the association of hepatitis B and cholangiocarcinoma was shown because of the endemicity of hepatitis B in both countries [26].

The association between diabetes, heavy alcohol drinking, smoking, and cholangiocarcinoma is not well established. Although some studies have shown a relationship between heavy alcohol drinking and cholangiocarcinoma, the risk factor may still be related to the presence of cirrhosis as a result of heavy alcohol drinking [16, 29, 30].

4.1 Genetic implications

Genetic studies showed that polymorphism in genes, which codes for enzymes implicated in the metabolism of carcinogens, DNA repair, and inflammation, can be either pro-carcinogenic or anticarcinogenic. Mutations in oncogenes such as tumor-suppressing genes, p53, APC, and Bcl-2, have been found in biliary duct tumors, which include amplification and overexpression of c-erbB-2 seen in cancers of the biliary tract. Mutations in K-ras, c-myc, c-neu, c-erbB-2, and c-met oncogenes have also been implicated, although mutations of RAS and TP53 genes are the most common abnormalities identified. Studies have shown that intrahepatic cholangiocarcinoma expresses CK7, CK19, and BerEP4 with cytoplasmic staining for CEA, unlike hepatocellular carcinoma. HER2/neu overexpression and high Ki-67 proliferation index are seen frequently in patients with nodal metastasis, as well as patients with reduced immunoexpression of E-cadherin. The suppressor p53 protein is involved in transcription, DNA repair, cell cycling, and genomic integrity. Three types of mechanisms of p16 inactivation have been reported in biliary neoplasms: deletion and point mutations of the p16INK4A gene and hypermethylation of 5′ regulatory regions of p16INK4A. It appears that the vascular endothelium growth factor expression is more in patients with extrahepatic cholangiocarcinoma [31–37].

4.2 Clinical presentation

Patients with hilar CC present with progressive obstructive jaundice earlier because of the location of the bile duct confluence; jaundice occurs even when the tumor is comparably small. Symptoms include malaise, weight loss, anorexia, nausea, vomiting, pruritus, and right upper quadrant pain. In patients with hilar CC, intrahepatic bile ducts are dilated, the gallbladder is usually not palpable, and the common duct is often collapsed on cholangiogram or ultrasound. In contrast, patients with carcinoma in the distal common bile duct or cystic duct present usually with a distended gallbladder and significant dilatation of the proximal bile duct system.

The symptoms are often obscure and many times ignored, making it difficult for early detection. As the tumor grows and obstructs the common hepatic duct and biliary confluence, jaundice gradually develops. Most patients with hilar cholangiocarcinoma seek medical advice because of progressive painless jaundice, accompanied with pruritus with multiple skin excoriations, clay-colored stool, and dark urine. Only patients with acute cholangitis present with fever, and this is seen only in 10% of the cases. On physical examination the liver is enlarged and firm. The gallbladder is usually impalpable, except in cases of distal biliary obstruction unlike hepatic biliary confluence obstruction where the gallbladder is not palpable [38, 39, 97].

4.3 Differential diagnosis

Biliary tumors are accompanied with painless jaundice which is suggestive of biliary obstruction. Although in the clinical findings, laboratory values such as tumor markers are non-specific and cannot specifically identify the exact cause of the stricture, differentiating extrahepatic biliary tumor from other causes of obstructive jaundice is important since the treatment is different.

4.4 Benign and malignant lesions masquerading as cholangiocarcinoma

Because of the close anatomic relationship of the biliary confluence to the gallbladder, carcinoma of the gallbladder may in some cases involve the hepatic hilum. Systemic dissemination of malignant melanoma can involve the biliary tract mimicking bile duct tumor. Neuroendocrine tumors can also involve the biliary tree. Lymph node metastatic cancers of the GI tract can also invade the bile duct as well as primary hematolymphoid malignancies which can affect the hepatic hilum [40–56]. Other legions include primary sclerosing cholangitis, secondary sclerosing cholangitis syndromes (portal biliopathy and AIDS cholangiopathy), inflammatory pseudotumor (autoimmune pancreatocholangitis), recurrent pyogenic cholangitis, Mirizzi syndrome (Type I–IV), biliary adenomas, hepatobiliary sarcoidosis, xanthogranulomatous cholecystitis and cholangitis, chemotherapy-induced sclerosing cholangitis [40–56].

5. Pathology

5.1 Gross appearance

Macroscopic appearance of CC of the extrahepatic bile ducts can be grouped into three types, sclerosing/scirrhous, nodular, or papillary. Sclerosing/scirrhous tumors are the most common. They may also be a combination "nodular sclerosing." Papillary variant accounts for 10% of all CC, most commonly seen in the distal bile duct but may also be present in hilus [57].

5.2 Pre-malignant lesions

Biliary adenoma: Although these are benign tumors, a small proportion may progress to carcinoma. Papillomatosis: Because of its multicentricity, it has a greater malignant potential and, whenever it is encountered, complete excision. Although difficult it is highly recommended.

Biliary cyst adenoma: Dysplastic changes leading to malignant transformation can occur with cysto-adenocarcinoma [24, 25].

5.3 Variants

Adenocarcinoma is the most common accounting for 90%, about two-third of all such tumors; it shows some focal intestinal differentiation with goblet and neuroendocrine cells. Variants include intestinal type, papillary adenocarcinoma, and mucinous adenocarcinoma. Overall, papillary adenocarcinoma has better prognosis even with lymph node metastasis. The mucinous adenocarcinoma produces an abundance of mucin secretion. Perineural and neural invasion is common. Clear cell carcinoma, hepatic carcinoma, and signet ring carcinoma are all variants of cholangiocarcinoma. Carcinosarcoma can be differentiated from squamous carcinoma because of the presence of spindle cell in the sarcoma variant. Some of these tumors can be keratinizing, while others are not. Small-cell carcinomas are endocrine tumors with varying degrees of differentiation; synaptophysin and chromogranin are necessary to confirm their endocrine nature [57].

6. Staging

In accordance with the American Joint Committee on Cancer (AJCC), the staging of extrahepatic cholangiocarcinoma is based on the extent of the primary tumor (T stage), extent of regional lymph node involvement (N stage), and presence of distant metastasis (M stage) (**Table 1**). An alternative to staging system proposed by Bismuth and Corlette classifies cholangiocarcinoma, based on the location of the tumor with respect to the hilum and on the extent of ductal involvement (**Figure 1**). AJCC staging is based largely on pathologic criteria and has little clinical significance since most patients present with T3 (stage IVA) tumors based on invasion of the liver. This neither says much about its resectability nor does it correlate with survival. In the AJCC system, patients with involved N1 and N2 lymph nodes are

Anatomic stage/prognostic groups			
Stage 0	Tis	N0	M0
Stage I	T1	N0	M0
Stage II	T2a-b	N0	M0
Stage IIIA	T3	N0	M0
Stage IIIB	T1-3	N1	M0
Stage IVA	T4	N0-1	M0
Stage IVB	AnyT	N2	M0
	AnyT	Any N	M1
Primary tumor (T)			
TX	Primary tumor cannot be assessed		
T0	No evidence of primary tumor		
Tis	Carcinoma in situ		
T1	Tumor confined to the bile duct, with extension up to the bile duct, with extension up to the muscle layer or fibrous tissue		
T2a	Tumor invades beyond the wall of the bile duct to surrounding adipose tissue		
T2b	Tumor invades adjacent hepatic parenchyma		
T3	Tumor invades unilateral branches of the portal vein or hepatic artery		
T4	Tumor invades main portal vein or its branches bilaterally or the common hepatic artery or the second-order biliary radicals bilaterally or unilateral second-order biliary radicals with contralateral portal vein or hepatic artery involvement		
Primary tumor (T)			
NX	Regional lymph nodes cannot be assessed		
N0	No regional lymph node metastasis		

N1	Regional lymph node metastasis (including nodes along the cystic duct, common bile duct, hepatic artery, and portal vein)
N2	Metastasis to periaortic, pericaval, superior mesenteric artery, and celiac artery lymph nodes
Distant metastasis (M)	
M0	No distant metastasis
M1	Distant metastasis

Table 1.
American Joint Committee on Cancer Seventh edition TNM staging for perihilar bile duct cancer. Anatomic stage/prognostic groups

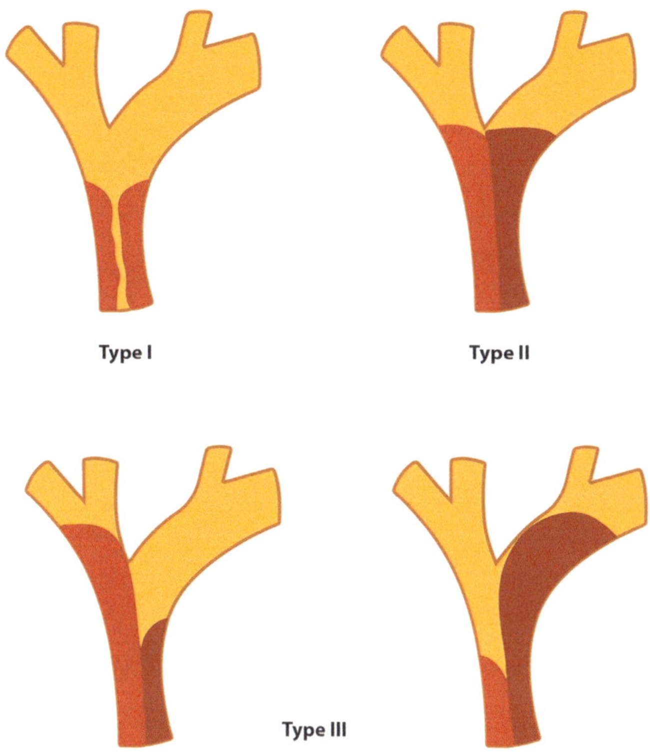

Figure 1.
Original Bismuth-Corlette classification.

inappropriately staged the same, since patients with metastatic disease to N2 lymph nodes (celiac, periduodenal, or retroperitoneal) are not candidates for resection and should be considered to have M1 disease. The Bismuth-Corlette system is more clinically relevant if not too simplified, but it also correlates poorly with resectability and survival. The Japanese Society of Biliary Surgery (**Table 2**) established a separate pathological staging system. In this system, the T classification is meticulously divided into categories of invasion because of its histological landmarks such as mucosa, serosa, and subserosa and its depth of invasion to adjacent structures such as the liver or pancreas which is classified into less than 5 mm, between 5 and 20 mm, and greater than 20 mm. Vascular invasion is distinguished between portal and hepatic artery, with each type having three depths (adventitial, tunica medial, and tunica intimal with stenosis or obstruction) numbered 1–3, respectively. This

pT classification				
pT	**Contents**			
pT1	m, fm, hinf0, panc0, pv0, a0			
pT2	ss, hinf1, panc1, pv0, a0			
pT3	se, hinf2, panc2, pv1, a1			
pT4	si, hinf3, panc3, pv2, pv3, a2, a3			
Lymph node grouping				
Lymph node (site number)	**Group**			
	Hilar and proximal	**Middle**	**Distal**	
Infrapyloric LN (6)	pN3	pN3	pN3	
LN around the common hepatic artery (8)	pN2	pN2	pN2	
LN at the splenic hilum (10)	pN3	pN3	pN3	
LN along the splenic artery (11)	pN3	pN3	pN3	
LN at the hepatic hilum (12 h)	pN1	pN2	pN2	
LN along the hepatic artery (12a)	pN1	pN2	pN2	
Periportal LN (12p)	pN1	pN2	pN2	
Pericholedochal LN (12b)	pN1	pN1	pN1	
LN around the cystic duct (12c)	pN1	pN1	pN1	
Posterior superior pancreaticoduodenal LN (13a)	pN2	pN2	pN2	
Posterior inferior pancreaticoduodenal LN (13b)	pN3	pN3	pN3	
LN along the superior mesenteric artery (14)	pN3	pN3	pN2	
Para-aortic LN (16)	pN3	pN3	pN3	
Anterior superior pancreaticoduodenal LN (17a)	pN3	pN3	pN3	
Anterior inferior pancreaticoduodenal LN (17b)	pN3	pN3	pN3	

Stage grouping	**H(−) and P(−) and M(−)**				**H(+) and/or P(+)**
					and/or
	pN0	**pN1**	**pN2**	**pN3**	**M(+) and any N**
pT1	I	II	III	IVa	IVb
pT2	II	III	III	IVa	IVb
pT3	III	III	IVa	IVb	IVb
pT4	IVa	IVa	IVb	IVb	IVb

Table 2.
Japanese Society of Biliary Surgery classification for cholangiocarcinoma.

classification is not popular outside of Japan due to its lack of complexity and authenticity. The Bismuth-Corlette system has since then modified its classifications (**Figure 2**) from its original: Type I, non-obstructed primary confluence; Type

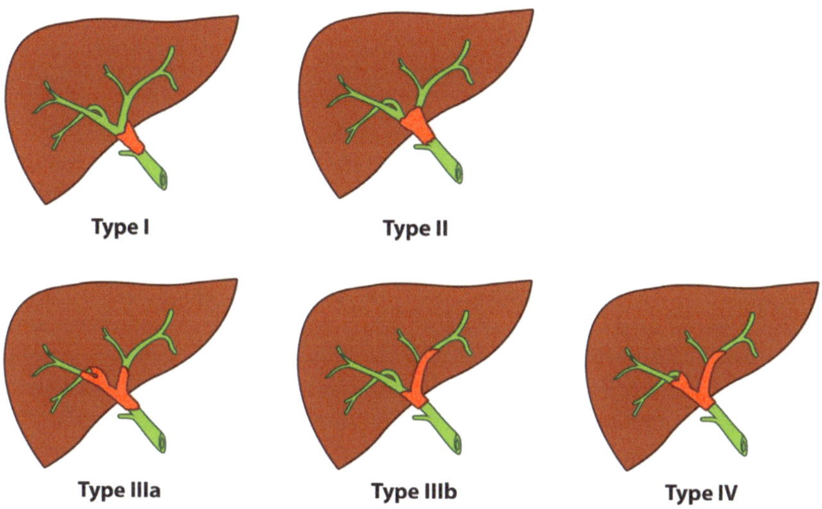

Figure 2.
Modified Bismuth-Corlette classification. Type I, tumor entirely below the confluence; Type II, tumors affecting the confluence; Type III, tumors occluding the confluence extending to the first-order right (IIIa) or left (IIIb) intrahepatic ducts; Type IV, involving both hepatic ducts or are multicentric.

II, obstruction limited to primary confluence; Type III, primary confluence with extension to the right or left secondary confluence; and Type IV, extension involving bilateral biliary ductal systems.

6.1 Bismuth-Corlette classification

None of the current staging systems takes into account local factors such as vascular invasion and hepatic lobar atrophy, which are important determinants for resectability and surgical outcome.

The TNM system can only be determined postoperatively and on final pathological specimen. A modified preoperative T staging was proposed by Jarnagin/Blumgart (**Table 3**). In this staging, the nodal and distal metastases are not considered. Going from T1 to T3, the nodal and distal metastasis increases. In their series, resectability was 59% with T1 and 0% with T3. Negative resection margin, concomitant hepatic resection, and well-differentiated tumor are independent predictors of long-term survival. With the Jarnigan/Blumgart system, a more in-depth framework was utilized to base preoperative decisions by predicting not only resectability but also the likelihood of R0 resection and subsequent survival.

Stage	Criteria
T1	Tumor involving biliary confluence ± unilateral extension to second-order biliary radicles
T2	Tumor involving biliary confluence ± unilateral extension to second-order biliary and ipsilateral portal vein involvement ± ipsilateral hepatic atrophy
T3	Tumor involving biliary confluence ± bilateral extension to second-order biliary radicles or unilateral extension to second-order biliary radicles with contralateral portal vein involvement or unilateral extension to second-order biliary radicles with contralateral hepatic lobar atrophy or main or bilateral portal venous involvement

Table 3.
Blumgart preoperative T staging system

7. Investigation and diagnosis

7.1 Evaluation of liver functional status

Liver function test and Child-Pugh score (MELD score).

Radiological: computer tomography volumetric analysis, hepatic steatosis measurement.

Some centers have taken into consideration the bioenergetics which includes the redox state of hepatocyte mitochondrial by quantifying the amount of ketone bodies in the serum of the patient, as well as the measurement of cellular energy charge through the measurement of AMP, ADP, ATP which can correlate with the phosphorylation ability of the hepatocytes. An abnormal functioning hepatocyte will have an alteration in energy level. Another emmerging technique is the magnetic resonance spectroscopy which is an in vivo non-invasive measurement of intracellular metabolism in relationship to phosphorylation. Other tests, such as dynamic studies (clearance tests, e.g., indocyanine green, aminopyrine, MEGX, hexose sugar handling capacity, hepatic scintigraphy, and portal vein embolization) [58].

7.2 Role of tumor markers

There seems to be no specific screening for Cholangiocarcinoma that is effective accept the laboratory values which may indicate obstructive cholestasis with hyper bilirubinemia and elevated alkaline phosphatase. The levels of CA 19-19, CEA, and CA-125 may be elevated, but only CA 19-9 is sensitive and specific 79% and 98% at the cut off value of 129 units/ml. Tumor markers are helpful when used together with other diagnostic tests. CA 19-9, CEA, and CA-125, may be elevated in patients with cholangiocarcinoma. CA 19-9 is less sensitive in patients with PSC, 53% at a cut off of greater than 100 units/L and usually would be undetectable in some patients lacking blood type Lewis antigen who usually do not produce CA 19-9. Patients lacking blood-type Lewis antigen (10%) do not produce CA 19-9. CA 19-9 are non-specific because they are also elevated in other gastrointestinal tumors. CEA alone has a low sensitivity and specificity for the diagnosis of cholangiocarcinoma. Siquiera and his associates demonstrated in their study that CEA > 5.2 ng/mL in combination with CA 19-9 > 180 U/ml had a sensitivity of 100% and a specificity of 78.4% for the detection of cholangiocarcinoma in patients with PSC.

However, Patel et al. compared the levels of CA 19-9 in 36 patients with cholangiocarcinoma without PSC. They found a cutoff value of CA 19-9 > 100 units/ml with a sensitivity of 53% for the diagnosis of cholangiocarcinoma and a true negative rate of 76% for nonmalignant liver diseases and 92% for benign biliary stricture. All the studies show, in patients with PSC, CA 19-9 has a cutoff value of >100 U/ml and a sensitivity of 75–89% while a specificity of 80–86% for the detection of cholangiocarcinoma. Newer markers, such as the human mucin subtypes A and C (mucin-5 AC), trypsinogen, and soluble fragment of cytokeratin 19, are currently being investigated, although Bamrungphon et al. reported that mucin-5 AC at a cutoff value of 0.074 had a sensitivity of 71% and a specificity of 90% for the diagnosis of CC. In another study of tumor stage resectability, CA 19-9 and CEA levels increased significantly with rising tumor stages. Patients with preoperative serum levels of CA 19-9 (> 1000 U/ml) and CEA (>14.4 ng/ml) showed a significant poorer resectability rate [59, 60].

8. Imaging

The most commonly used imaging modalities are ultrasound, CT scan, MRI/MRCP, direct cholangiogram, and PET scan.

Ultrasound usually shows dilatation of the biliary tree either intra- or extrahepatic biliary tree. Distal obstruction is associated with both extra- and intrahepatic dilatation, whereas proximal obstruction is associated with intrahepatic dilatation. It can show the extent of the tumor involvement as well as encroachment to the portal vein. Contrast-enhanced ultrasound is currently being used in the diagnosis of hilar cholangiocarcinoma. Endoscopic ultrasound is valuable in assessing patients with cholangiocarcinoma and its involvement with neighboring structures, especially the middle and distal part of the bile duct, but it cannot distinguish between benign and malignant lesions [61, 62]. CT scan with intravenous contrast scanning plays an important role in the diagnosis and staging of hilar cholangiocarcinoma, since it can provide information regarding the location of biliary obstruction, tumor extension, vascular invasion, hepatic lobar atrophy, lymph node involvement, distant metastases, and encroachment of the portal vein. It is even more accurate when high-resolution multidetector-row CT scanners are used [63]. The combination of MRI with MRCP is another effective imaging modality for staging of hilar cholangiocarcinoma. Like CT scanning, MRI provides reliable information regarding the level of biliary obstruction, vascular invasion, hepatic lobar atrophy, lymph node involvement, as well as distant metastases. Unlike PTC, MRCP is not invasive. It has an accuracy of 72–83% [64, 65]. ERCP and PTC involve injection of contrast into the biliary tree. They are commonly used in the preoperative diagnosis. It is unreliable in patients with complete bile duct obstruction. It seems to be a simple procedure but could be met with some complications, which include bile leakage, cholangitis, bleeding, pancreatitis, and duodenal perforation. Mortality rate ranges between 0.6 and 5.6%. Because of its limitation it has been replaced with MRCP [64]. FDG-PET is not superior to conventional triple-phase CT scanning in the detection of primary lesion of hilar cholangiocarcinoma. However, it is more accurate than conventional CT scan in detecting distant metastases with a sensitivity between 56 and 100% and a specificity of 88% [66].

9. Tissue analysis

Endoscopic-guided fine-needle aspiration is useful when the results of brush cytology and forceps biopsy are inconclusive; EUS-guided FNA can be done. Its negative predictive value is 29%, which means that a negative EUS-guided FNA does not necessarily exclude the possibility of hilar CC [62].

Although the diagnosis of hilar cholangiocarcinoma is primarily based on imaging, it has its limitation because of its inability to differentiate between benign and malignant strictures. Brush cytology and forceps biopsy via ERCP or PTC are the most frequently used modality for pathological diagnosis. With brush cytology most of the time the tissue obtained may not be sufficient to make a good pathological assessment because the tumor may be hidden within fibrous stroma allowing for a lower sensitivity as opposed to forceps biopsy [67]. The FISH assay can identify malignant cells by its fluorescent probes as well as detecting abnormal chromosomes in the biliary cells obtained by brush cytology. It is a very advanced technique and when complemented with DIA which identifies malignant cells by the use of special stains that quantify nuclear DNA as well as demonstrate aneuploidy are both promising [68]. The exfoliative cells found in the bile can further be analyzed in the contest of its DNA methylation status, thereby demonstrating evidence of malignancy in patients with equivocal findings, such as biliary stricture. The most well studied are P16 and APC gene [69].

10. Treatment of cholangiocarcinoma

Only surgical excision of all detectable tumors is associated with an improvement in 5-year survival. However, surgery can only cure a minority of patients, with a 20–30% 5-year survival for distal lesion and a 9–18% 5-year survival for proximal lesions. The management of patients with CC should be a multidisciplinary approach. Patients' general physical condition must be assessed, including pulmonary and cardiovascular function, nutritional, extent of cholestasis, and a proper assessment of resectability as well as future liver remnant. Preoperative staging must have been done and resectability is assessed. The following criteria would suggest an irresectable tumor: involvement of bilateral second-order intrahepatic or extra hepatic ducts, or multifocal tumor on cholangiography, extensive involvement of the main portal vein, involvement of major vessels or ducts on the contralateral side of the liver, liver atrophy, and nodal metastasis to N2 lymph nodes (peripancreatic, periduodenal, celiac, superior mesenteric, or posterior pancreaticoduodenal lymph nodes). Lymph node involvement and peritoneal seeding may be difficult to detect preoperatively. In this case, laparoscopy and laparoscopic ultrasound offer additional benefit. Laparoscopy includes likelihood of visualizing small metastatic tumor deposits on the surface of the liver and peritoneum, which would otherwise go undetected. Laparoscopic staging avoids extensive preparation for inoperable patients. Cytological analysis of peritoneal washings can be done during laparoscopy.

11. Is there a role of preoperative optimization of the liver prior to surgical resection?

Jaundice is usually the presenting symptom in patients with hilar cholangiocarcinoma, even when the tumor is small. Complete tumor clearance may require extensive liver resection to obtain long-term survival. Having said that, extensive liver resection has a mortality rate of up to 20% and morbidity rates of up to 67%. Parenchymal transection in a jaundice and cholestatic liver may result in increased bleeding, biliary fistula, sepsis, and impaired liver regeneration. In attempting to improve preoperative outcome, many centers have advocated preoperative biliary drainage and ipsilateral portal vein embolization of the hemiliver to be resected, to improve the future of the liver remnant. In a recent French national study, serum bilirubin was found to be correlated with mortality, which ranged from 9 to 27% when serum bilirubin was more than 300 units (French International Value). The choice of the route for biliary drainage is controversial. Endoscopic approach is often difficult in patients with complete obstruction, especially when the left duct requires drainage. Percutaneous transbiliary drainage can be done either unilateral or bilateral. But most centers prefer a unilateral PTBD on the side of the future liver remnant. It takes about 4–6 weeks prior to surgery and normalization of serum bilirubin. Note that preoperative biliary drainage resulted in an increase of postoperative infectious complication rates [70, 71]. Although there is no randomized study to show the benefit of portal vein embolization in hilar cholangiocarcinoma, some people argue in favor of PVE, especially when extended right lobe resection and vascular reconstruction are anticipated since resection of more than 60% of the total liver volume may result in postoperative liver failure [72].

12. Surgical treatment

It is important to determine whether an R0 resection is achievable. Is the future liver remnant sufficient for patient survival? Is there distant metastasis and involvement of level 3 lymph nodes, celiac, SMA, and aortocaval, which precludes curative resection [73, 74]? In the last 20 years, extended liver and bile duct resection has become the standard of care for hilar cholangiocarcinoma. In general, a remnant liver consistent of 20–30% of the total liver mass is sufficient to prevent liver failure following resection as long as this remaining portion is not compromised. To accomplish this, it might be necessary to employ volumetric studies performed by radiologists of the total and future remnant liver. Some centers advocate the use of (ICG) 15-min retention rate and ICG clearance (K-value).

Peritoneal carcinomatosis and small intrahepatic metastasis are often not detectable by conventional preoperative investigations. This has motivated the use of staging laparoscopy and an analysis of peritoneal washing for patients with HCCA [75].

12.1 Is there a role of local resection in biliary cholangiocarcinoma?

Local resection is not an adequate curative operation for HCCA, except perhaps for small papillary Klatskin tumor without bile duct confluence involvement (Type I Bismuth-Corlette classification, TIs and T1 AJCC staging) [76].

The goal of the surgical principle in the management of HCCA is to accomplish a RO resection, not only cancer-free proximal and distal margin but also cancer-free margins around the hepatoduodenal ligament. Patients should undergo a thorough surgical exploration, especially if they have no preoperative signs of metastasis or locally unresectable disease, because despite the selectivity and specificity of ultrasonography, CT scan, and MRI, almost 45% of patients who are explored are found to have peritoneal tumor seedings, lymph node involvement, liver metastasis, or advanced disease, all of which preclude resection. These patients may benefit with biliary bypass and cholecystectomy to prevent future occurrence of acute cholecystitis.

At laparotomy, a generous Kocher maneuver is performed to mobilize the pancreatic head. During this procedure, hepatoduodenal ligament, retropancreatic and celiac arteries are also exposed. Distal bile duct is isolated and resected at its intrapancreatic portion. Distal margin should be submitted for intraoperative frozen section examination. If the frozen section is negative, the distal stump is closed. If the distal margin is positive for cancer, then a concomitant pancreaticoduodenectomy is indicated. This applies to resectable tumors. For unresectable perihilar malignant lesions, Roux-en-Y choledocojejunostomy to either segment II or III bile ducts or the right hepatic duct can be performed.

For curative lesions, the location and local tumor involvement determine the extent of resection. Perihilar tumors involving the bifurcation or above the common hepatic duct (BC Type I or II) without any vascular involvement may be a candidate for local resection with portal lymphadenectomy, cholecystectomy, common bile duct excision, and bilateral Roux-en-Y hepaticojejunostomy. For lesions involving the right or left duct (Bismuth-Corlette IIIa and IIIb), right or left hepatic lobectomy can be performed. Distal bile duct tumors are frequently resectable, and if resectable they are treated with pylorus-preserving pancreatoduodenectomy, whereas in unresectable distal bile duct tumors, Roux-en-Y hepaticojejunostomy, cholecystectomy, and gastrojejunostomy should be performed to prevent gastric outlet obstruction as the tumor progresses. The principal caudate lobe duct drains into the left hepatic duct. Tumors extending into the left hepatic duct almost always involve the caudate duct and will usually necessitate caudate resection. Also, a dilated caudate duct may be suggestive of tumor involvement. The lobe is involved by HCCA in 40–98% of patients. Retrospective studies have shown a decrease in local recurrence and improvement in 5-year survival with concomitant caudate resection. Tsao et al. stated that combining hilar resection and partial hepatectomy with complete caudate lobe resection can be performed safely. Others consider removing the caudate lobe, only when the left hepatic duct is involved.

Depending on the level of ductal involvement with surrounding structures the following procedures can be performed:

Left or right hepatectomy with caudate lobectomy is performed for tumor involving the left or right secondary biliary duct. Resection of the caudate lobe along with left or right hepatectomy or sectionectomy is no more controversial in our center. We recommend mandatory caudectomy irrespective of the type of procedure to be carried on. Extended left or right hepatectomy with caudate lobectomy can be considered depending on the extent of biliary and parenchymal involvement. For B/C, Type IV tumors which involve bilateral secondary biliary radicles are considered unresectable. These patients are candidates for palliative treatment or liver transplantations. In various series of Klatskin tumors, portal vein involvement has been found in 16–22% of patients. In addition, its propensity to spread along the bile duct and nerves, that accompany the hepatic and celiac arteries, as well as its direct spread to lymph nodes (53%) and adjacent liver parenchyma, has made it difficult to achieve an R0 resection with removal of the duct alone [73].

Central hepatectomy is indicated for tumors located at the confluence of the three segments deep within the liver substance in patients with good hepatic reserve. This involves removal of segment 4a, 4b, 5, and 8 [77, 78].

Ex situ ex vivo autotransplantation. This highly skilled bench surgery which involves total hepatectomy under hypothermic perfusion and complex reconstruction and reimplantation should only be attempted in experienced centers on carefully selected patients [79]. Bilioenteric continuity is essential to restore the continuity of bilioenteric flow. Mucosal to mucosal anastomosis is made between a Roux-en-Y loop of jejunum.

The role of lymphadenectomy in the staging is important, but its role in treatment is debatable. Although earlier studies showed its advantage, clinical evidence of the survival benefits of lymphadenectomy during extended resection remains low [80, 81]. Portal vein resection can be done in cases where the tumor is adherent to the portal vein. It is evident that combined portal vein resection offers improved survival when compared to no resection or a resection with positive margins. Portal vein resection for HCCA in experienced hands is not debatable and can be done, and sometimes the resected portal vein is replaced with autologous vein or interposition graft. However, hepatic artery involvement by the tumor previously was considered contraindication to resection but recently, some centers are resecting and reconstructing the hepatic artery for tumors involving secondary biliary radicles and hepatic artery. Hepatic artery reconstruction is an evolving technique, in which more studies must be done before it becomes a standard [82, 83].

12.2 Transplantation

Surgical R0 resection is clearly the definitive choice for patients with HCCA/ICCA and should be considered in all patients who are surgical candidates presenting with resectable tumors. Earlier studies of long-term survival outcome with the radical resection of early stage hilar tumor report a 5-year survival rate of 34%; the outcome for CCA with aggressive features such as tumor size more than 2 cm multifocality remains poor because of limitation of resection as treatment modality in achieving clear margins. For ICCA, the 5-year survival rate with negative surgical margins approached 31%; there are no survivors with residual disease. The median time for recurrence ranges from 9 to 20 months, with the most common site being the liver remnant, occurring in 38–70% of cases and metastasis to the regional lymph node, lung, and bones. Unfortunately many HCCA and ICCA tumors are considered unresectable because of tumor extension to the hepatic parenchyma, major hepatic artery, and vein of both right and left hemilivers and metastasis to regional lymph nodes. Considering these circumstances for locally advanced HCCA/ICCA in the absence of distant metastasis, a total hepatectomy followed with regional lymphadenectomy followed by orthotopic liver transplantation offers a viable treatment option because it will address all relevant resection margins, as well as liver disease. Liver transplantation offers the advantage of removing all structures that may be involved by hilar cholangiocarcinoma including portal vein, bilateral hepatic duct, atrophic liver lobes, and hepatic artery. Total hepatectomy will permit R0 resection for locally advanced tumors which are beyond the ordinary criteria for resection using partial hepatectomy. Unfortunately early reports of transplantation in patients with cholangiocarcinoma were not successful, the 5-year survival was 20–30%, and it was considered a relative contraindication to liver transplantation. It was not until the group from the Mayo Clinic developed a protocol with the intent of treating a highly selected group of patients with CC.

The inclusion criteria involves a strict selection of patients with early stage HCCA either deemed locally unresectable or arising in the setting of underlying PSC. Patients with HCCA were included only if there was no mass lesion below the level of the cystic duct. The upper limit of tumor size was 3 cm. When the mass was visible in cross-sectional imaging studies, and there must be no evidence of intrahepatic or extrahepatic metastasis by any imaging studies, the initial protocol excluded patients with intrahepatic CC or gallbladder cancer (**Table 4**). Surgical intervention and percutaneous biopsy were avoided to minimize percutaneous seeding; candidates must have no active infection or medical condition to preclude neoadjuvant therapy or liver transplantation. The candidates underwent endoscopic ultrasound-guided regional lymph node aspiration before neoadjuvant therapy. Any patient with positive lymph node metastases are disqualified from subsequent liver transplantation. In the Mayo Clinic protocol, patients received external beam radiotherapy and transcatheter radiation with iridium (Ir) 192 through a wire placed endoscopically. Systemic 5-FU is given during radiation followed by oral capecitabine after radiation until the day of surgery. Before transplantation all

Variables	Mayo Clinic	UCLA
Hilar CC	Yes	Yes
Hilar CC size	<3 cm	<3 cm
Intrahepatic CC	No	Yes
Intrahepatic CC size	—	≤8 cm
Metastasis to hepatic parenchyma	Absent	Present or absent
Metastasis to regional lymph node	Absent	Present or absent
Metastasis to distant organ	Absent	Absent

Table 4.
Comparison of inclusion criteria for Mayo Clinic and UCLA treatment protocol of cholangiocarcinoma.

patients undergo a staging laparotomy, including a biopsy of at least one lymph node along the proper hepatic artery and another along the common bile duct, as well as any suspicious lymph node. Only those with negative lymph nodes will proceed with transplantation. The results of transplantation showed 1- and 5-year survival rates of 91 and 76%, respectively, and 5 year recurrence-free survival rate of 60%. Predictors for tumor recurrence in older patients include CA 19-9 levels over 100 units/mL on the day of transplantation, prior cholecystectomy, tumor grade, and residual greater than 2 cm, as well as perineural invasion in explant. A multicenter study showed a 2- and 5-year recurrence-free survival of 78 and 65%, respectively. There is a significant morbidity associated with this, such as cholangitis, intrahepatic abscess and sepsis, infection, and tumor necrosis from chemoradiation. The greatest concern is vascular complication after transplantation. The overall vascular complication rate after transplantation was 41%; 21% of patients developed hepatic arterial complications, whereas 20% experienced portal venous complications. To avoid using irradiated native hepatic artery, an infrarenal interposition arterial graft was routinely used to reconstruct arterial inflow in all deceased donor grafts, whereas the native hepatic artery was used in live donor grafts. Although the Mayo Clinic protocol has resulted in excellent long-term recurrence-free survival, proponents for expansion of OLT criteria argue that patient inclusion guideline restricted to hilar tumors based only on size may exclude patients with locally advanced hilar CC stage IIA, IIB, and III (AJCC). Despite absence of metastatic disease, Hong et al. have recently reported that survival benefits can also be achieved in patients with locally advanced CC (>3 cm in size, tumor extension to hepatic parenchyma, branches of portal vein or hepatic artery, presence of perineural and lymphovascular invasion). Using a neoadjuvant and adjuvant protocol, they had a 5-year disease recurrence-free survival of 47% in patients who received OLT in combination with neoadjuvant and adjuvant therapies than 0% in the resection group [84–86].

12.3 Is there a role of adjuvant therapy in the treatment of cholangiocarcinoma?

Some centers reported the use of intraoperative radiotherapy, Busse et al. These results are rather conflicting with no significant difference in mean survival. Although Kamada et al. suggested that radiotherapy may increase survival in patients with positive hepatic duct resection margins. If this modality is to be used postoperatively, metal clips should be placed to mark the area of the anastomosis after resection or areas of known or suspected residual tumors. Despite significant advances in the surgical management of perihilar cholangiocarcinoma, the only chance for long-term survival remains complete resection with negative margins. Radiation therapy alone has no significant impact in prolonging survival in these patients. Some centers are using gemcitabine in combination with cisplatin along with radiation, although anecdotal but rather promising. Both gemcitabine and cisplatin have been demonstrated in recent years to have activity against hilar CC, and a recent phase 3 trial suggests that the best results can be achieved with a combination of these two agents [87–91].

12.4 Palliative therapy

Most patients with HCCA may not be suitable for surgical resection. If a patient is considered irresectable after histological or cytological tissue is confirmed to be cancerous, palliative measures can be an option. The palliative measures include biliary decompression either surgical, endoscopic, or percutaneous techniques which can be applied in unresectable tumors as well as chemotherapy, radiation therapy, and photodynamic therapy. Palliative biliary bypass can be performed by exposing the left hepatic duct; this involves (1) opening the umbilical fissure, elevating the base of the segment 4 lobe, while lowering the left hepatic ductal system from the undersurface of the quadrate lobe, (2) exposing branches of the left duct by dissection at the base of the ligamentum teres, (3) by partial excision of the left lateral segment and performing a biliary-enteric anastomosis to the opening in branches of the left hepatic duct (Longmire procedure), and (4) Cahow's intrahepatic cholangiojejunostomy. If the left hepatic duct is not accessible, the right drainage system (V or VI) can be exposed by a hepatotomy at the base of the gallbladder fossa, but in general, segment III bypass is performed, unless the left liver is atrophic or is heavily involved with tumors or in cases of the primary lesion extending to the umbilical fissure of the liver [92, 93].

12.5 What are the importance of endoscopic and percutaneous methods and when is it indicated?

The use of these modalities differs from center to center. Routine biliary drainage is not recommended before assessing resectability, except in patients with suppurative cholangitis or patients with severe renal dysfunction and malnutrition. Endoscopic palliation of jaundice in patients with HCCA is best achieved in patients in whom preoperative drainage was achieved endoscopically. At the present time, percutaneous drainage of the biliary system is a useful tool in patients in whom endoscopic drainage cannot be achieved due to technical difficulties and in non-availability of advanced endoscopic facilities. Endoscopic stent insertion can also be used to deliver other forms of palliative adjuvant therapy, such as brachytherapy and photodynamic therapy. The development of newer stents and techniques for deployment as well as the rapidly emerging applications of EUS could widen the scope of endoscopy as a palliative tool in HCCA. It is technically easier to place endoscopically or percutaneously in patients with distal lesions than proximal lesions. The patency for metallic stents at the hilar region is less than those placed in the distal duct. Endoscopic, percutaneous, and operative approaches to biliary decompression are effective. The patency for distal stent is higher than the proximal stents. It might be technically difficult to place a stent to the proximal lesion endoscopically. In this scenario, percutaneous approach may be better for proximal lesions. Stents can be placed unilateral or bilateral and sometimes unilateral stent placement may be adequate. The patency of self-expanding bare metal stents is higher than polyethylene plastic stents. Covered stents have a comparable patency rate to bare metal stents, but they are associated with an increased rate of complication which involves stent migration. Photodynamic therapy is emerging as a promising option for palliative therapy, while brachytherapy is still evolving. Both approaches remain, at this time, investigational for CC palliation. It is important that the optimal management of patients with CC requires a multidisciplinary team of clinicians, including surgeons, interventional and diagnostic radiologists, gastroenterologist, and hepatologists [94, 95].

12.6 Photodynamic therapy and immunotherapy

This approach has been used as a palliative measure for tumors of the esophagus, colon, and stomach. It is promising as a means of providing biliary decompression without stents or another means of treating those with microscopically involved bile duct margins. It uses two nontoxic components, a photosensitizing chemical called photosensitizer and light which is applied in sequence. The wavelength of the photosensitizer corresponds to the absorption spectra of the photosensitizer, and it is activated by several wavelengths. To achieve tumor necrosis, it is better to use the photosensitizer with the longest wavelength. With oxygen molecules present, this results in the release of various cytotoxic species, like singlet oxygen and other reactive oxygen species. Photodynamic therapy is both anti-angiogenic which damages tumor endothelial cells as well as dose-dependent immune responses. At high doses, it causes damage to the cellular membranes and the blood vessel which leads to recruitment of neutrophils and monocytes/macrophages and activation of pro-inflammatory cytokines like interleukin IL-1beta, IL-2, and tumor necrosis factor TNF-alpha. This results in the enhancement of the host immune system which plays an important role in secondary cytotoxicity and tumor control. Serum IL-6, a bile duct epithelium growth factor correlating with tumor burden in CC, decreases after PDT. The side effect of PDT is cutaneous photosensitivity [96]. Although not conclusive, but at its preliminary stage as discussed earlier, biliary cancers that express epidermal growth factor and angiogenesis have been correlated with poor prognosis. Erlotinib and EGFR tyrosine kinase inhibitor and bevacizumab, a vascular endothelial growth factor (VEGF) inhibitor, have been shown to have activity in biliary cancer. Inhibitors of epidermal growth factor receptor family, such as erlotinib, cetuximab, and lapatinib, were recently investigated. Furthermore, bortezomib (an inhibitor of proteasome), imatinib mesylate (an inhibitor of c-kit-R), bevacizumab (an inhibitor of VEGF), and sorafenib (a multiple kinase inhibitor), that blocks not only tyrosine kinase but also serine/threonine kinases along the RAS/RAF/MEK/ERK pathway, have been used. Early evidence of antitumor activity was seen, but the results are still too early and require further investigation [36].

13. Summary

Cholangiocarcinoma is a very deadly disease, which if diagnosed early and if the patient is subjected to a complete surgical resection may have an impact in long-term survival. Having said that, much progress has been made with multidisciplinary services, transplantation, aggressive surgical approach, and hopefully with new developments in technology and research; we hope to improve the survival rate.

Author details

Samuel Romeo Obiekwe[1*], Nathaly Suzett De La Roca[2] and Jean Saric[3]

1 Huntington Park Hospital, Los Angeles, USA

2 University of California, San Diego, USA

3 Department of Surgery, University of Bordeaux, France

*Address all correspondence to: sobiekwe@yahoo.com

References

[1] Taylor-Robinson SD, Foster GR, Arora S, et al. Increase in primary liver cancer in the UK, 1979–94. Lancet. 1997; **350**:1142-1143

[2] Patel T. Increasing incidence and mortality of primary intrahepatic cholangiocarcinoma in the United States. Hepatology. 2001;**33**:1353-1357

[3] Klatskin G. Adenocarcinoma of the hepatic duct at its bifurcation within the porta hepatis: An unusual tumor with distinctive clinical and pathological features. The American Journal of Medicine. 1965;**38**:241-256

[4] Strasberg SM. Resection of hilar cholangiocarcinoma. HPB Surgery. 1998;**10**:415

[5] Zimmerman A. Tumors of the bile ducts-pathological aspects. In: Blumgart LH, editor. Surgery of the Liver and Biliary Tract. 3rd ed. Vol. 200. London: W.B. Saunders. pp. 953-975

[6] Renard P, Boutron MC, Faivre J, et al. Biliary tract cancers in Cote d'Or (France): Incidence and natural history. Journal of Epidemiology and Community Health. 1987;**41**:344-348

[7] Shahip Y, El-Sharag HB. The epidemiology of cholangiocarcinoma. Seminars in Liver Disease. 2004;**24**: 115-124

[8] Khan SA, Taylor-Robinson SD, Toledano MD, et al. Changing international trends in mortality rates for liver, biliary and pancreatic tumors. Journal of Hepatology. 2002;**37**:806-813

[9] Shaib YB, Davila JA, McGlynn K, et al. Rising incidence of intrahepatic cholangiocarcinoma in the United States: A true increase? Journal of Hepatology. 2004;**40**:472-477

[10] Blechacz BR, Gores GJ. Cholangiocarcinoma. Clinics in Liver Disease. 2008;**12**(1):131-150

[11] van Kaick G, Wesch H, Luhrs H, et al. Neoplastic diseases induced by chronic alpha-irradiation—Epidemiological, biophysical, and clinical results of the German Thorotrast Study. Journal of Radiation Research (Tokyo). 1991;**32**(Suppl. 2):20-33

[12] LaRusso NF, Shneider BL, Black D, et al. Primary sclerosing cholangitis: Summary of a workshop. Hepatology. 2006;**44**(3):746-764

[13] Kaewpitoon N, Kaewpitoon SJ, Pengsaa P, et al. *Opisthorchis viverrini*: The carcinogenic human liver fluke. World Journal of Gastroenterology. 2008;**14**(5):666-674

[14] Upatham ES, Vivyant V. *Opisthorchis viverrini* and opisthorchiasis: A historical review and future perspective. Acta Tropica. 2003; **88**(3):171-176

[15] Lee CC, Wu CY, Chen GH. What is the impact of coexistence of hepatolithiasis on cholangiocarcinoma? Journal of Gastroenterology and Hepatology. 2002;**17**:1015-1020

[16] Donato F, Gelatti U, Tagger A, et al. Intrahepatic cholangiocarcinoma and hepatitis C and B virus infection, alcohol intake, and hepatolithiasis: A case-control study in Italy. Cancer Causes & Control. 2001;**12**(10):959-964

[17] Kobayashi S, Asano T, Yamaski M, et al. Risk of bile duct carcinogenesis after excision of extrahepatic bile ducts in pancreaticobiliary maljunction. Surgery. 1999;**126**(5):939-944

[18] Watanabe Y, Toki A, Todani T. Bile duct cancer developed after cyst

excision for choledochal cyst. Journal of Hepato-Biliary-Pancreatic Surgery. 1999;**6**(3):207-212

[19] Soreide K, Korner H, Havnen J, et al. Bile duct cysts in adults. The British Journal of Surgery. 2004;**91**(12): 1538-1548

[20] Edil BH, Cameron JL, Reddy S, et al. Choledochal cyst disease in children and adults: A 30-year single institution experience. Journal of the American College of Surgeons. 2008;**206**(5): 1000-1005

[21] Mabrut JY, Bozio G, Hubert C, et al. Management of congenital bile duct cysts. Digestive Surgery. 2010;**27**(1): 12-18

[22] Ohta T, Nagakawa T, Ueno K, et al. Clinical experience of biliary tract carcinoma associated with anomalous union of the pancreatic ductal system. The Japanese Journal of Surgery. 1990; **20**:36-43

[23] Tocchi A, Mazzoni G, Liotta G, et al. Late development of bile duct cancer in patients who had biliary-enteric drainage for benign disease: A follow-up study of more than 1,000 patients. Annals of Surgery. 2001;**234**:210-214

[24] Callea F, Sergi C, Fabbretti G, et al. Precancerous lesions of the biliary tree. Journal of Surgical Oncology. Supplement. 1993;**3**:131-133

[25] O'Shea M, Fletcher HS, Lara JF. Villous adenoma of the extrahepatic biliary tract: A rare entity. The American Surgeon. 2002;**68**:889-891

[26] Yamamoto S, Kubo S, Hai S, et al. Hepatitis C virus infection as a likely etiology of intrahepatic cholangiocarcinoma. Cancer Science. 2004;**95**(7):592-595

[27] El-Serag HB, Engels EA, Landgren O, et al. Risk of hepatobiliary and pancreatic cancers after hepatitis C virus infection: A population-based study of U.S. Veterans. Hepatology. 2009;**49**(1):116-123

[28] Sorensen HT, Friis S, Olsen JH, et al. Risk of liver and other types of cancer in patients with cirrhosis: A nationwide cohort study in Denmark. Hepatology. 1998;**28**(4):921-925

[29] Shaib YH, El-Serag HB, Nooka AK, et al. Risk factors for intrahepatic and extrahepatic cholangiocarcinoma: A hospital-based case-control study. The American Journal of Gastroenterology. 2007;**102**(5):1016-1021

[30] Shaib YH, El-Serag HB, Davila JA, et al. Risk factors for intrahepatic cholangiocarcinoma in the United States: A case-control study. Gastroenterology. 2005;**128**(3):620-626

[31] Grainge MJ, West J, Solaymani-Dodaran M, et al. The antecedents of biliary cancer: A primary care case-control study in the United Kingdom. British Journal of Cancer. 2009;**100**(1): 178-180

[32] Prawan A, Kukongviriyapan V, Tassaneeyakul W, et al. Association between genetic polymorphisms of CYP1A2, arylamine N-acetyltransferase 1 and 2 and susceptibility to cholangiocarcinoma. European Journal of Cancer Prevention. 2005;**14**(3): 245-250

[33] Khan SA, Thomas HC, Toledano MB, et al. p53 mutations in human cholangiocarcinoma: A review. Liver International. 2005;**25**:704-716

[34] Liu XF, Zhang H, Zhu SG, et al. Correlation of p53 gene mutation and expression of p53 protein in cholangiocarcinoma. World Journal of Gastroenterology. 2006;**12**:4706-4709

[35] Zheng J, Zhu YM. Expression of c-erbB-2 proto-oncogene in extrahepatic

cholangiocarcinoma and its clinical significance. Hepatobiliary & Pancreatic Diseases International. 2007;**6**:412-415

[36] Yoshikawa D, Ojima H, Iwasaki M, et al. Clinicopathological and prognostic significance of EGFR, VEGF, and HER2 expression in cholangiocarcinoma. British Journal of Cancer. 2008;**98**: 418-425

[37] Guedj N, Zhan Q, Perigny M, et al. Comparative protein expression profiles of hilar and peripheral hepatic cholangiocarcinomas. Journal of Hepatology. 2009;**51**:93-101

[38] Sitzmann J, Greene P. Perioperative predictors of morbidity following hepatic resection for neoplasm. Annals of Surgery. 1994;**219**:13-17

[39] Noun R, Jagot P, Farges O, et al. High preoperative serum alanine transferase levels: Effect on the risk of liver resection in child grade A cirrhotic patients. World Journal of Surgery. 1997;**21**:390-395

[40] Are C, Gonen M, DAngelica M, et al. Differential diagnosis of proximal biliary obstruction. Surgery. 2006;**140**: 756-763

[41] Dasgupta T, Brasfield R. Metastatic melanoma: A clinicopathologic study. Cancer. 1964;**15**:1323-1339

[42] El Rassi ZS, Mohsine RM, Berger F, et al. Endocrine tumors of the extrahepatic bile ducts: Pathological and clinical aspects, surgical management and outcome. Hepato-Gastroenterology. 2004;**51**:1295-1300

[43] Riopel MA, Klimstra DS, Godellas CV, et al. Intrabiliary growth of metastatic colonic adenocarcinoma: A pattern of intrahepatic spread easily confused with primary neoplasia of the biliary tract. The American Journal of Surgical Pathology. 1997;**21**:1030-1036

[44] Van Slyck EJ, Schuman BM. Lymphocytic lymphosarcoma of the gallbladder. Cancer. 1972;**30**:810-816

[45] Broome U, Olsson R, Loof L, et al. Natural history and prognostic factors in 305 Swedish patients with primary sclerosing cholangitis. Gut. 1996;**38**: 610-615

[46] Abdalian R, Heathcote EJ. Sclerosing cholangitis: A focus on secondary causes. Hepatology. 2006;**44**: 1063-1074

[47] Sasahira N, Kawabe T, Nakamura A, et al. Inflammatory pseudotumor of the liver and peripheral eosinophilia in autoimmune pancreatitis. World Journal of Gastroenterology. 2005;**11**:922-925

[48] Sperling RM, Koch J, Sandhu JS, et al. Recurrent pyogenic cholangitis in Asian immigrants to the United States: Natural history and role of therapeutic ERCP. Digestive Diseases and Sciences. 1997;**42**:865-871

[49] Nash JA, Cohen SA. Gallbladder and biliary tract disease in AIDS. Gastroenterology Clinics of North America. 1997;**26**:323-335

[50] Kim KP, Kim MH, Song MH, et al. Autoimmune chronic pancreatitis. The American Journal of Gastroenterology. 2004;**99**:1605-1616

[51] Sarin SK, Bhatia MU. Portal biliopathy in extrahepatic portal vein obstruction. Indian Journal of Gastroenterology. 1992;**2**:A82

[52] Johnson LW, Sehon JK, Lee WC, et al. Mirizzi's syndrome: Experience from a multi-institutional review. The American Surgeon. 2001;**67**:11-14

[53] Kawakatsu M, Vilgrain V, Zins M, et al. Radiological features of papillary adenoma and papillomatosis of the biliary tract. Abdominal Imaging. 1997; **22**:87-90

[54] Cox CE, Davis-Allen A, Judson MA. Sarcoidosis. The Medical Clinics of North America. 2005;**89**:817-828

[55] Howard TJ, Bennion RS, Thompson JE Jr. *Xanthogranulomatous cholecystitis*: A chronic inflammatory pseudotumor of the gallbladder. The American Surgeon. 1991;**57**:821-824

[56] Batts KP. Ischemic cholangitis. Mayo Clinic Proceedings. 1998;**73**: 380-385

[57] Albore-Saavedra J, Scoazec JC, Wittekind C, et al. Carcinoma of the gallbladder and extrahepatic bile ducts. In: Hamilton SR, Aaltonen LA, editors. World Health Organization Classification of Tumours. Tumors of the Digestive System. Lyon: International Agency for Research on Cancer Press; 2000. pp. 206-214

[58] Jiao L, El-Desoky A, Seifalian A, et al. Effect of liver blood flow and function on hepatic indocyanine green clearance measured directly in a cirrhotic animal model. The British Journal of Surgery. 2000;**87**:568-574

[59] Alvaro D. Serum and bile biomarkers for cholangiocarcinoma. Current Opinion in Gastroenterology. 2009;**25**:279-284

[60] Bamrungphon W, Prempracha N, Bunchu N, et al. A new mucin antibody/enzyme-linked lectin sandwich assay of serum MUC5AC mucin for the diagnosis of cholangiocarcinoma. Cancer Letters. 2007;**247**:301-308

[61] Sharma MP, Ahuja V. Aetiological spectrum of obstructive jaundice and diagnostic ability of ultrasonography: A clinician's perspective. Tropical Gastroenterology. 1999;**20**:167-169

[62] Fritscher-Ravens A, Broering DC, Knoefel WT, et al. EUS-guided fine-needle aspiration of suspected hilar cholangiocarcinoma in potentially operable patients with negative brush cytology. The American Journal of Gastroenterology. 2004;**99**:45-51

[63] Akamatsu N, Sugawara Y, Osada H, et al. Diagnostic accuracy of multidetector-row computed tomography for hilar cholangiocarcinoma. Journal of Gastroenterology and Hepatology. 2010; **25**:731-737

[64] Park HS, Lee JM, Choi JY, et al. Preoperative evaluation of bile duct cancer: MRI combined with MR cholangiopancreatography versus MDCT with direct cholangiography. AJR. American Journal of Roentgenology. 2008;**190**:396-405

[65] Park MS, Kim TK, Kim KW, et al. Differentiation of extrahepatic bile duct cholangiocarcinoma from benign stricture: Findings at MRCP versus ERCP. Radiology. 2004;**233**:234-240

[66] Fritscher-Ravens A, Bohuslavizki KH, Broering DC, et al. FDG PET in the diagnosis of hilar cholangiocarcinoma. Nuclear Medicine Communications. 2001;**22**:1277-1285

[67] Weber A, von Weyhern C, Fend F, et al. Endoscopic transpapillary brush cytology and forceps biopsy in patients with hilar cholangiocarcinoma. World Journal of Gastroenterology. 2008;**14**: 1097-1101

[68] Baron TH, Harewood GC, Rumalla A, et al. A prospective comparison of digital image analysis and routine cytology for the identification of malignancy in biliary tract strictures. Clinical Gastroenterology and Hepatology. 2004;**2**:214-219

[69] Yin XY, Yan G, Peng JX, et al. The clinical values of methylation status of P16, APC genes in bile in diagnosis of malignant obstructive jaundice. In: Gastrointestinal Cancer Symposium

Proceedings; San Francisco, California, USA; 2011. p. 91

[70] Grandadam S, Compagnon P, Arnaud A, et al. Role of preoperative optimization of the liver for resection in patients with hilar cholangiocarcinoma type II. Annals of Surgical Oncology. 2010;**17**:3155-3161

[71] Nagino M, Takada T, Miyazaki M, et al. Preoperative biliary drainage for biliary tract and ampullary carcinomas. Journal of Hepato-Biliary-Pancreatic Surgery. 2008;**15**:25-30

[72] Hwang S, Lee SG, Ko GY, et al. Sequential preoperative ipsilateral hepatic vein embolization after portal vein embolization to induce further liver regeneration in patients with hepatobiliary malignancy. Annals of Surgery. 2009; **249**:608-616

[73] Nagino M, Nimura Y, Hayakawa N, et al. Logistic regression and discriminant analyses of hepatic failure after liver resection for carcinoma of the biliary tract. World Journal of Surgery. 1993;**17**:250-255

[74] Jarnagin WR, Fong Y, DeMatteo RP, et al. Staging resectability, and outcome in 225 patients with hilar cholangiocarcinoma. Annals of Surgery. 2001;**234**:507-519

[75] Weber SM, DeMatteo RP, Fong Y. et al, Staging laparoscopy in patients with extrahepatic biliary carcinoma. Analysis of 100 patients. Annals of Surgery. 2002;**235**:392-399

[76] Capussotti L, Vigano L, Ferrero A, et al. Local surgical resection of hilar cholangiocarcinoma: Is there still a place? HPB: The Official Journal of the International Hepato Pancreato Biliary Association. 2008;**10**(3):174-178

[77] Hadjis NS, Blenkharn JI, Alexander N, et al. Outcome of radical surgery in hilar cholangiocarcinoma. Surgery. 1990;**107**(6):597-604

[78] Neuhaus P, Jonas S, Bechstein WO, et al. Extended resections for hilar cholangiocarcinoma. Annals of Surgery. 1999;**230**(6):808-818; discussion 19

[79] Pichlmayr R, Bretschneider HJ, Kircchner E, et al. Ex-situ operation an der Leber. Eine neue Moeglichkeit in der Leber chirugie. Langenbecks Archiv für Chirurgie. 1988;**373**(2):122-126

[80] Bismuth H, Nakache R, Diamond T. Management strategies in resection for hilar cholangiocarcinoma. Annals of Surgery. 1992;**215**:31-38

[81] Kitagawa Y, Nagino M, Kamiya J, et al. Lymph node metastasis from hilar cholangiocarcinoma: Audit of 110 patients who underwent regional and paraaortic node dissection. Annals of Surgery. 2001;**233**:385-392

[82] Nagino M, Nimura Y, Nishio H, et al. Hepatectomy with simultaneous resection of the portal vein and hepatic artery for advanced perihilar cholangiocarcinoma: An audit of 50 consecutive cases. Annals of Surgery. 2010;**252**:115-123

[83] Hemming AW, Mekeel K, Khanna A, et al. Portal vein resection in the management of hilar cholangiocarcinoma. Journal of the American College of Surgeons. 2011; **212**(4):604-613; discussion 613-6

[84] Mantel HT, Rosen CB, Heimbach JK, et al. Vascular complications after orthotopic liver transplantation after neoadjuvant therapy for hilar cholangiocarcinoma. Liver Transplantation. 2007;**13**:1372-1381

[85] Rea DJ, Heimbach JK, Rosen CB, et al. Liver transplantation with neoadjuvant chemoradiation is more effective than resection for hilar

cholangiocarcinoma. Annals of Surgery. 2005;**242**:451-458; discussion 8-61

[86] Hong JC, Jones CM, Duffy JP, et al. Comparative analysis of resection and liver transplantation for intrahepatic and hilar cholangiocarcinoma: A 24-year experience in a single center. Archives of Surgery. 2011;**146**:683-689

[87] Deziel DJ, Kiel KD, Kramer TS, et al. Intraoperative radiation therapy in biliary tract cancer. American Journal of Surgery. 1988;**54**:402-407

[88] McMasters KM, Tuttle TM, Leach SD, et al. Neoadjuvant chemoradiation for extrahepatic cholangiocarcinoma. American Journal of Surgery. 1997;**174**: 605-609

[89] Pitt HA, Nakeeb A, Abrams RA, et al. Perihilar cholangiocarcinoma. Postoperative radiotherapy does not improve survival. Annals of Surgery. 1995;**221**:788-797; discussion 797-8

[90] Busse PM, Stone MD, Sheldon TA, et al. Intraoperative radiation therapy for biliary tract carcinoma: Results of a 5-year experience. Surgery. 1989;**105**: 724-733

[91] Kamada T, Saitou H, Takamura A, et al. The role of radiotherapy in the management of extrahepatic bile duct cancer: An analysis of 145 consecutive patients treated with intraluminal and/ or external beam radiotherapy. International Journal of Radiation Oncology, Biology, Physics. 1996;**34**: 767-774

[92] Traynor O, Castaing D, Bismuth H. Left intrahepatic cholangio-enteric anastomosis (round ligament approach): An effective palliative treatment for hilar cancer. The British Journal of Surgery. 1987;**74**:952-954

[93] Jagannath P, Bhansali MS, Desouza LJ, et al. Palliative segment III biliary bypass (left cholangio-jejunostomy) in malignant block at porta hepatis. Indian Journal of Gastroenterology. 1992;**11**: 71-72

[94] Abraham NS, Barkun JS, Barkun AN. Palliation of malignant biliary obstruction: A prospective trial examining impact on quality of life. Gastrointestinal Endoscopy. 2002; **56**(6):835-841

[95] Nordback IH, Pitt HA, Coleman J, et al. Unresectable hilar cholangiocarcinoma: Percutaneous versus operative palliation. Surgery. 1994;**115**:597-603

[96] Huang Z, Xu H, Meyers AD, et al. Photodynamic therapy for treatment of solid tumor potential and technical challenges. Technology in Cancer Research & Treatment. 2008;7:309-320

[97] Tsao J, Nimura Y, et al. Management of hilar cholangiocarcinoma. Annals of Surgery. 2000;**323**(2):166-174